Applying Nursing Process

A Step-By-Step Guide

Rosalinda Alfaro-LeFevre, MSN, RN is president of Teaching Smart/Learning Easy in Stuart, Florida. An established and successful author, she is known for making difficult topics easy to understand. As a result, her work has been translated into five languages. With more than 20 years of clinical practice and teaching experience in both baccalaureate and associate degree nursing programs, she has a wealth of nursing expertise to draw upon, whether writing, consulting, or leading seminars.

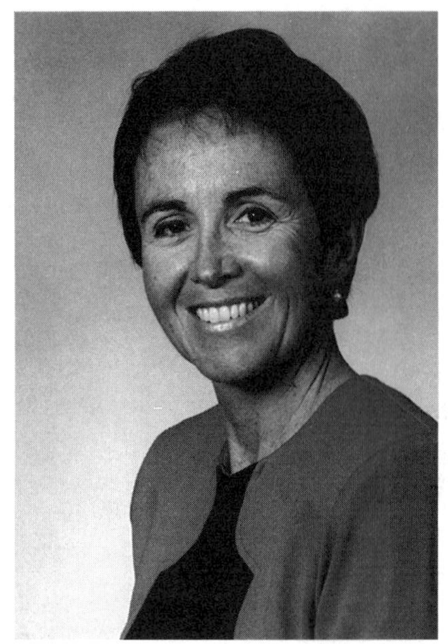

Applying Nursing Process

A Step-By-Step Guide

4th Edition

Rosalinda Alfaro-LeFevre, MSN, RN
President
Teaching Smart/Learning Easy
Stuart, Florida

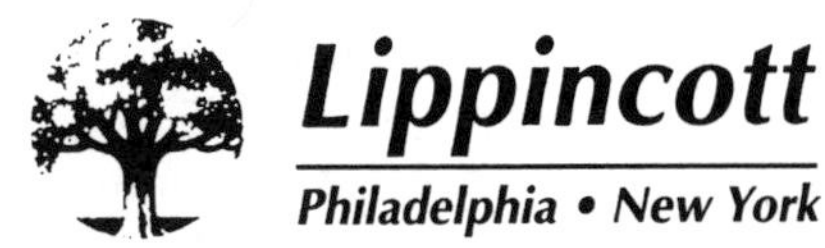

Sponsoring Editor: Susan M. Keneally
Associate Managing Editor: Barbara Ryalls
Senior Production Manager: Helen Ewan
Production Coordinator: Sharon McCarthy
Assistant Art Director: Kathy Kelley-Luedtke
Indexer: Lynn Mahan

Edition 4

9 8 7 6 5 4 3

Library of Congress Cataloging-in-Publication Data

Alfaro-LeFevre, Rosalinda.
Applying nursing process : a step-by-step approach / Rosalinda Alfaro-LeFevre.—4th ed.
p. cm.
Includes bibliographical references and index.
ISBN 0-397-55453-2 (alk. paper)
1. Nursing—Handbooks, manuals, etc.
I. Title. [DNLM: 1. Nursing Process. WY 100 A385a 1998]
RT51.A6255 1998
610.73—DC21
DNLM/DLC
for Library of Congress 97-25194
CIP

Care has been taken to confirm the accuracy of the information presented and to describe generally accepted practices. However, the authors, editors, and publisher are not responsible for errors or omissions or for any consequences from application of the information in this book and make no warranty, express or implied, with respect to the contents of the publication.

The authors, editors and publisher have exerted every effort to ensure that drug selection and dosage set forth in this text are in accordance with current recommendations and practice at the time of publication. However, in view of ongoing research, changes in government regulations, and the constant flow of information relating to drug therapy and drug reactions, the reader is urged to check the package insert for each drug for any change in indications and dosage and for added warnings and precautions. This is particularly important when the recommended agent is a new or infrequently employed drug.

Some drugs and medical devices presented in this publication have Food and Drug Administration (FDA) clearance for limited use in restricted research settings. It is the responsibility of the health care provider to ascertain the FDA status of each drug or device planned for use in their clinical practice.

Dedication

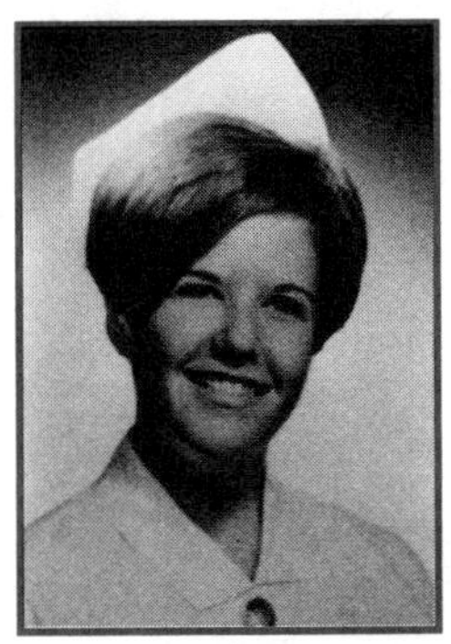

In Memory of Constance S. Sechrist, RN

March 10, 1948–December 27, 1995

It was Connie's choice to become a nurse that led to her illness. Years before wearing protective gloves became routine, as a junior student, she contracted the hepatitis virus from a patient. It's believed that same virus damaged her pancreas, causing diabetes and, eventually, complications (vision problems, heart disease, and kidney failure).

It was Connie's spirit and choice to become a nurse that enabled her to live each day to the max. Unlike a lawyer, who can't take care of her own legal needs, Connie was the best nurse she ever had. She could separate herself from "Connie, the patient" and go through the steps that "Connie the nurse" needed to do to keep herself going.

Contributor

Nancy Flynn, RNC, MSN
Clinical Nurse Educator
Bryn Mawr Hospital
Bryn Mawr, PA

Consultants/Review Board

Ella R. Anaya, RN, MSN
Sophomore Chair
Kent State University
Kent, OH

Ledjie Ballard, RN, MSN, CRNA
Consultant For Perioperative Processes & Systems Management
Seattle, WA

Cheryl L. Brady, RN, MSN
Assistant Nursing Professor
Kent State University
East Liverpool Campus
East Liverpool, OH

Lynda Juall Carpenito, RN, MSN, FNPC
President
LJC Consultants
Mickleton, NJ
Family Nurse Practitioner
Ches-Penn Community Health Center
Chester, PA

Carol Ann Coltrin
Associate Professor
Ventura College
Ventura, CA

Carol Hutton, EdD, ARNP
President
Hutton Associates
Boca Raton, FL

Bonnie Eyeler, MSN, RN, JD
Boca Raton, FL

Pauline McKinney Green, PhD, RN
Associate Professor
Howard University College of Nursing
Washington, DC

Sharon Johnson, MSN, RNC, CNA
Director of Clinical Practice/Outcome Management
Jefferson Home Health/Main Line Hospitals
Bryn Mawr, PA

Judith H. Lewis, EdD, RN
Director, Baccalaureate Program
St. Louis University School of Nursing
St. Louis, MO

Ainslie T. Nibert, RN, MSN, CCRN
Assistant Professor and BSN Department Chair
College of Nursing
Houston Baptist University
Houston, TX

Terri Patterson, RN, MSN, CRRN
President
Nursing Consultation Services LTD and LifeTrak LTD
Norristown, PA

Rebecca Resh, MEd
Coordinator of Licensing and Accrediting
Mediplex Rehabilitation Center
Camden, NJ

Carl Ross, RN, MSN
Clinical Instructor
Duquesne University
Pittsburgh, PA

Carol Taylor, CSFN, RN, MSN
PhD Candidate
Assistant Professor and Ethicist
School of Nursing
Georgetown University
Washington, DC

Toni C. Wortham, RNC, MSN
Professor
Madisonville Community College
Madisonville, KY

Elements Used to Promote Critical Thinking and Enhance Motivation to Learn*

1. Objectives written at the cognitive level of analysis precede each chapter.
2. Advance organizers and chapter overviews precede content.
3. Relevant terms are defined in the glossary, and more difficult terms are clarified in the text by definition, discussion, and use within context.
4. Illustrations are placed throughout to establish relationships and clarify text.
5. Analogies, examples, and case studies are used to clarify information and demonstrate relevance of content.
6. Rationales are highlighted in guidelines and displays, and integrated as needed in other parts of the text.
7. Questioning at the analysis level is used:
   - During content presentation to stimulate curiosity and give clues to what's important.
   - After the content (in Practice Sessions) to reinforce key points and provide the opportunity to test and refine knowledge.
8. Content is presented in such a way that those who need structure have it, without restricting those who require more creative freedom.
9. "Try This On Your Own" sessions are offered to allow for practice without concern about being evaluated by others.
10. Summaries (Key Points) are listed at the end of each chapter.

*References

Gearheart, B., Weishahn, M., & Gearheart, C. (1992). *The exceptional student in the regular classroom* (5th ed.). New York: Macmillan.

Ouellette, F. (1988). A textbook coding tool: Part 1, Assessing elements that promote analytic abilities. *Nurse Educator, 13*(5):8–13.

Ouellette, F. (1989). A textbook coding tool: Part 2, Assessing nursing textbooks. *Nurse Educator, 14*(1):19–22.

Preface

What's the Same About This Edition

Like the previous editions, this book is completely revised to reflect how the nursing process continues to evolve in a changing health care arena.

The overall goal is to provide a clear, concise presentation of the steps of the nursing process. Great pains have been taken to make this a user-friendly book that helps students use the nursing process effectively. Elements that promote critical thinking and enhance motivation to learn are integrated throughout (see facing page).

Principles and rules that provide a basis for making decisions and adapting to the constant changes in health care delivery are highlighted throughout. To help you master and apply content, you'll find practice sessions placed at strategic places in the reading. Example responses for practice sessions are found beginning on page 231.

The *Nursing Diagnosis Quick Reference Section* (beginning on page 193) provides easy access to information on all the diagnoses accepted for clinical testing by the North American Nursing Diagnosis Association.

Key Concepts Include:

- The role of knowledge, skills, and caring in demonstrating nursing process expertise (see figure on following page).
- The importance of mastering communication, interpersonal, and critical thinking skills.
- The importance of making changes early, based on assessment and reassessment, during *Implementation*, rather than waiting for a formal evaluation period.
- The significance of legal and ethical implications.
- The impact of cost containment and insurance requirements.

What's New About This Edition

This edition has been shortened and simplified, focusing on how to use the nursing process in various situations.

Greater Emphasis is Given to:

- Nurses' roles in homes, communities, and multidisciplinary practice.
- The shift in thinking from *diagnose and treat* to *predict, prevent, and manage*.
- The use of critical pathways and computers.
- How nurses' roles as diagnosticians and case managers continue to evolve.
- Cultural aspects of nursing care.

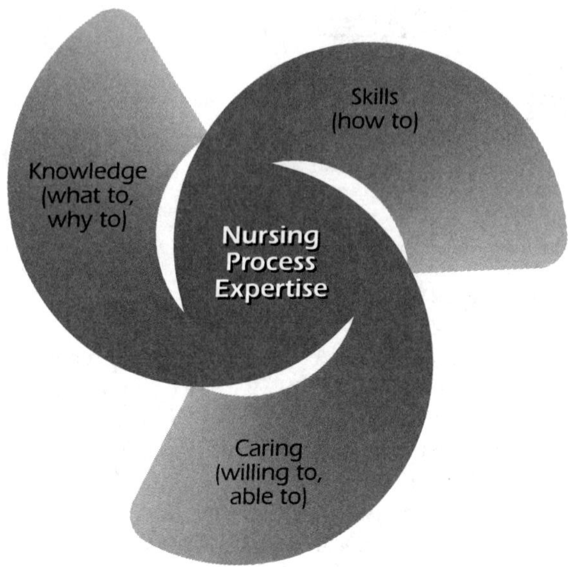

Other Changes Include:

- *What's in This Chapter?* precedes each chapter, giving a chapter synopsis.
- To stimulate thinking and reinforce content, "food for thought," labeled *Think About It* is integrated throughout.
- The Glossary and Bibliography have been moved to the back of the book.
- Appendices include an example critical path and listings of Nursing Interventions Classification (NIC) and Nursing Outcomes Classification (NOC).

A Word About "Patient/Client" and "He/She"

Whenever possible, I've used a fictitious name, or "someone," "person," "consumer," or "individual" instead of "client" or "patient" to help us keep in mind that each client or patient is an individual who has unique needs, values, perceptions, and motivations. "He" and "she" are used interchangeably to avoid the awkwardness of using he/she over and over.

Comments and Suggestions Welcomed

I welcome and appreciate suggestions for improvement—often the most significant changes are made based on student and faculty suggestions. Please direct mail to:

Rosalinda Alfaro-LeFevre, Author
Lippincott-Raven Publishers
c/o Nursing Editorial Department
227 East Washington Square
Philadelphia, PA 19106-3780
e-mail: r-alfaro@juno.com

Rosalinda Alfaro-LeFevre, MSN, RN

Acknowledgments

I want to thank my husband, Jim, for his love, support, and sense of humor and fun; and the rest of my family for being behind me all the way.

I also want to thank the following people for their belief in me and their contribution to my personal and professional growth: Louise and Nat Rochester, Heidi Laird, Ledjie Ballard, Annette Sophocles, Carol Taylor, Barbara Cohen, Lynda and Richard Carpenito, Mary Jo Boyer, John Payne, Charlie and Nancy Lindsay, Marty Kenney, Emily and Alex Barosse, Becky Resh, Diane Verity, Nancy Flynn, Carol Hutton, Bonnie Eyler, the Villanova University Nursing Faculty, and the past and present nurses at Paoli Memorial Hospital.

My special thanks go to: the Nursing Editorial division of Lippincott-Raven, especially to Susan Keneally, Assistant Editor, and Barbara Ryalls, Associate Managing Editor, who were able to stay focused on the details of this project, even when their desks were full of other priorities; and of course, the sales and marketing department whose efforts have helped make this book a bestseller.

Contents

Practice Sessions

CHAPTER 1

CHAPTER 2

CHAPTER 3

CHAPTER 4

CHAPTER 5

CHAPTER 6

Introduction

This book is intended to help make the nursing process make sense to you. I've purposely made the reading as easy as possible and used many real-life examples to make learning this material both interesting and relevant. I've also incorporated real-life situations into practice sessions that are specifically designed to give you the opportunity to become actively involved in using the steps of the nursing process.

It's my hope that you'll use this book in whatever way you find most helpful; for example, if you need added clarification, write it on the pages. Mark it up and make it yours. Do the practice sessions when you feel you need clarification or when reviewing for an exam—they're there for you to refine and test your knowledge. For quick feedback, example responses are in the back of the book (except for Try This on Your Own sessions, which, for the most part have no *right* answers because they present ways you can learn without the anxiety of being tested).

Applying Nursing Process

A Step-By-Step Guide

CHAPTER 1

Nursing Process Overview

OBJECTIVES

Once you complete this chapter, you should be able to:

- Describe the five steps of the nursing process.
- Explain the relationships among the steps of the nursing process.
- List at least four benefits of using the nursing process.
- Discuss how the nursing process complements what other disciplines (physicians, physical therapists, etc.) do.
- Describe three qualities required to be competent in using the nursing process.
- Determine five critical thinking characteristics you'd like to acquire or improve.
- Define critical thinking in nursing using your own terms.
- Identify behaviors that promote positive interpersonal relationships.
- Explain what it takes to be willing and able to care.
- Describe at least four caring behaviors.

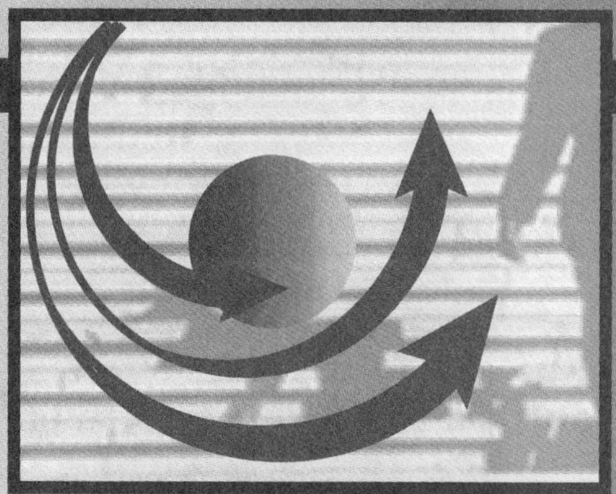

Practice Sessions

- **Practice Session I:** Steps of the Nursing Process
- **Practice Session II:** Critical Thinking, Interpersonal Skills, and Willingness and Ability to Care

What's in this chapter?

This chapter defines nursing process and addresses the question, "Why learn about it?" It then presents a short overview of each step of the nursing process and explains why the steps are interrelated and overlapping. Finally, it focuses on what it takes to be competent using the nursing process (knowledge, skills, and caring), and gives suggestions for how to develop critical thinking skills.

What Is the Nursing Process and Why Learn About It?

The nursing process is a systematic method of giving humanistic care that focuses on achieving desired outcomes (results) in a cost-effective fashion. It's *systematic* in that it consists of five steps—*Assessment, Diagnosis, Planning, Implementation,* and *Evaluation*—during which you take deliberate steps to maximize efficiency and attain long-term beneficial results. It's *humanistic* in that it's based on the belief that as we plan and deliver care, we must consider the unique interests, ideals, and desires of the health care consumer (person, family, community).

There are at least three major reasons for learning to use the nursing process: 1) Its use is a requirement set forth by national practice standards (see Display 1-1). 2) It provides the basis for questions on state board exams. 3) Its principles and rules are designed to promote critical thinking in the clinical setting.

The nursing process, as described in this book, is based on principles and rules that are known to promote efficient nursing care. If you take the time to learn and apply these principles you'll improve your ability to solve problems, make decisions, and maximize

DISPLAY 1-1 American and Canadian Standards of Practice Related to Nursing Process

American Nurses Association (ANA) Practice Standards*

Standards of Care (Use of Nursing Process)

I **Assessment:** The nurse collects client health data.
II **Diagnosis:** The nurse analyzes assessment data in determining diagnoses.
III **Outcome Identification:** The nurse identifies expected outcomes individualized to the client.
IV **Planning:** The nurse develops a plan of care that prescribes interventions to attain expected outcomes.
V **Implementation:** The nurse implements the interventions identified in the plan of care.
VI **Evaluation:** The nurse evaluates the client's *progress* toward attainment of outcomes.

Canadian Nurses Association (CNA) Standard II†

Standard II. Nursing practice requires the effective use of the nursing process.

Nurses are required in any practice setting to do the following: (1) collection of data, (2) analysis of data, (3) planning of the intervention, (4) implementation of the intervention, and (5) evaluation.

---

*From: *Standards of Clinical Practice* (1991). American Nurses Association. Washington, DC.

†Summarized from: Canadian Nurses Association (CNA) Standards for Nursing Practice prepared and revised by a Task Group to Develop a Definition of Nursing Practice and Standards for Nursing Practice. Ottawa, CNA, 1987.

opportunities and resources, and you'll form thinking habits that will help you pass state board exams. In the clinical setting, you'll have the satisfaction of achieving the ultimate goals* of nursing:

- To prevent illness and promote, maintain, or restore health (in terminal illness, to achieve a peaceful death)
- To enable people to manage their own health care
- To provide cost-effective, quality care
- To continue to find ways of improving satisfaction with health care delivery.

NOTE: If you don't understand a term, look it up in the glossary beginning on page 249. Throughout this book, the term **medical problem** refers to diseases or trauma diagnosed by physicians or advanced practice registered nurses (APRNs). APRNs have a wide scope of authority to act (may include treating some medical problems and prescribing some medications) by virtue of advanced credentials (usually completion of a master's program and certification). The term **medical order** refers to interventions prescribed by physicians or APRNs to treat medical problems.

Steps of the Nursing Process

Here's a brief description of the steps of the nursing process:

1. ***Assessment.*** You collect and examine information about health status, looking for evidence of abnormal function or risk factors that may contribute to health problems (eg, smoking). You also look for evidence of client strengths.
2. ***Diagnosis (Problem Identification).*** You analyze the data (information) and identify actual and potential problems, which are the basis for the plan of care. You also identify strengths, which are essential to developing an efficient plan.
3. ***Planning.*** Here, you do four key things:

   Determine immediate priorities: Which problems need immediate attention? Which ones can wait? Which ones will nursing focus on? Which ones will you delegate or refer to someone else? Which ones require a multidisciplinary approach?

   Establish expected outcomes (goals): Exactly what do you expect the patient or client to accomplish, and in what time frame?

   Determine interventions: What interventions (nursing actions) will you prescribe to achieve the outcomes?

* The terms *goal* and *outcome* are often used interchangeably. However, *outcome* is the preferred term when addressing what *the patient or client* is expected to accomplish (as compared to what the *nurse* is expected to accomplish). See in-depth discussion in Chapter 4 (page 120).

Record or individualize the plan of care. Will you write your own plan, or will you adapt a standard plan to meet your patient's specific situation?

4. ***Implementation.*** You put the plan into action—but you don't just *act*. You act thoughtfully:

   Assess the person's current status before acting. Are there any new problems? Has anything happened that requires an immediate change in the plan?

   Perform the interventions, monitoring the person carefully and making changes as needed. What's the response? Do you need to change something? You don't wait until the "formal" evaluation period to make changes if something needs changing today.

   Report and record. Are there any signs you must report immediately? What are you going to chart and where and how are you going to chart it?

5. ***Evaluation.*** You determine whether the desired outcomes have been achieved, whether the interventions were effective, and whether changes need to be made; then you change or terminate the plan as indicated.

   How does the person's health status compare with the expected outcomes? Is your patient able to do what you planned? If not, why? Are there new care priorities?

   If you achieved the outcomes, is the person ready to manage his care on his own? Do you need to make referrals for health promotion? What made the plan work? What could have been done to make things easier?

To remember the steps of the nursing process, remember the first letter of each of the steps (the mnemonic ADPIE [pronounced ad′pi]). Study Table 1-1, which summarizes the steps of the nursing process and compares them with those of the familiar problem-solving method.

TABLE 1–1 Nursing Process versus Problem-Solving Method

Nursing Process	Problem-Solving Method
Assessment: Continuously collecting data about health status to monitor for evidence of health problems and risk factors that may contribute to health problems (eg, smoking).	**Encountering a problem:** Collecting data about the problem.
Diagnosis: Analyzing data to identify actual and potential health problems and strengths.	**Analyzing data** to determine exactly what the problem is.
Planning: Determining desired outcomes (specific goals) and identifying interventions to achieve the outcomes.	**Making a plan** of action.
Implementation: Putting the plan into action and observing initial responses.	**Putting the plan into action.**
Evaluation: Determining how well the outcomes have been achieved and deciding whether changes need to be made.	**Evaluating results.**

Think About It

Each patient and family holds the key to effective nursing care. When you establish trust, provide information, and encourage people to take an active role in maximizing their ability to function, you empower them to achieve optimum health, and you open the door to patient satisfaction and health care efficiency.

Relationships Among the Steps of the Nursing Process

The steps of the nursing process are interrelated and overlapping as explained in the following section.

Assessment and Diagnosis

The first two steps, *Assessment* and *Diagnosis,* overlap significantly. As you gather information, you start to interpret what the information means, even though you haven't put the whole picture together yet. For example, you might be assessing someone and note an irregular pulse, swollen ankles, and difficulty breathing. It's likely that you'd begin to make a tentative diagnosis (this patient may have a heart problem) as you continue with the assessment.

The diagram below shows the close relationship between *Assessment* and *Diagnosis.*

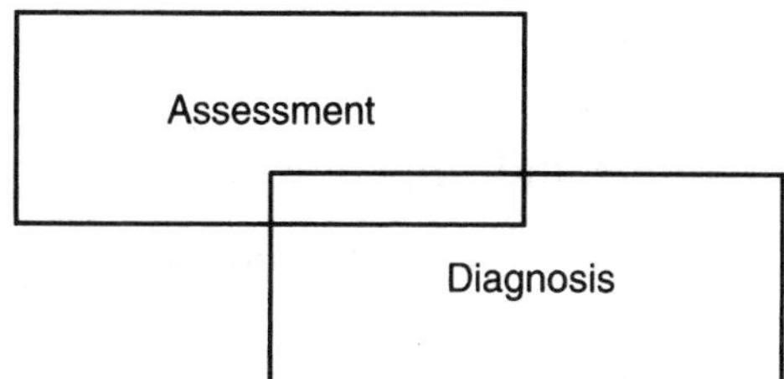

Diagnosis and Planning

Diagnosis is related to *Planning* for four reasons:

1. The outcomes you establish during *Planning* are derived directly from the problems you diagnose. For example, if you diagnose *Constipation,* you must determine an appropriate outcome for this problem (eg, "the person will have a soft bowel movement at least every other day").
2. The interventions you plan should be designed to achieve the expected outcomes and prevent, resolve, or control the problems you identify during *Diagnosis.* For example, for *Constipation,* you'd plan interventions to promote bowel regularity (eg, teaching the need for adequate hydration, dietary roughage, and so forth).

3. There are times when you have to act quickly, implementing a mental plan of action, before identifying all the problems. For example, if you encounter a life-threatening problem, take immediate action. Once the situation is under control, analyze all the data in more depth.
4. You need to incorporate the strengths you identify during *Diagnosis* into the plan. For example, if you learn someone is unable to plan meals but has relatives who are willing to help, you use the relatives as a resource (eg, teaching relatives how to include foods with high roughage).

The diagram below shows the relationship between *Diagnosis* and *Planning*.

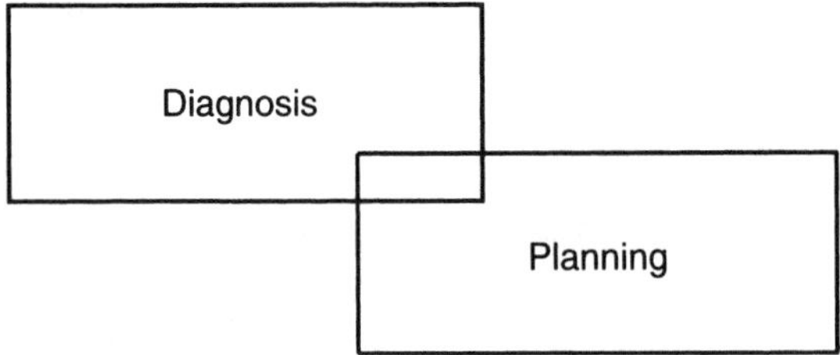

Think About It

If your diagnoses are inaccurate, incomplete, or vague, or if you haven't identified strengths, it's unlikely your plan will be effective or efficient. It may even be dangerous.

Planning and Implementation

Planning and *Implementation* are closely related and overlapping for two reasons.

1. The plan guides interventions performed during *Implementation*.
2. As already mentioned, there may be times when you have to plan and implement nursing actions quickly, before the entire plan is developed. And sometimes, for simple problems, you act without formal planning.

The diagram below shows the relationship between *Planning* and *Implementation*.

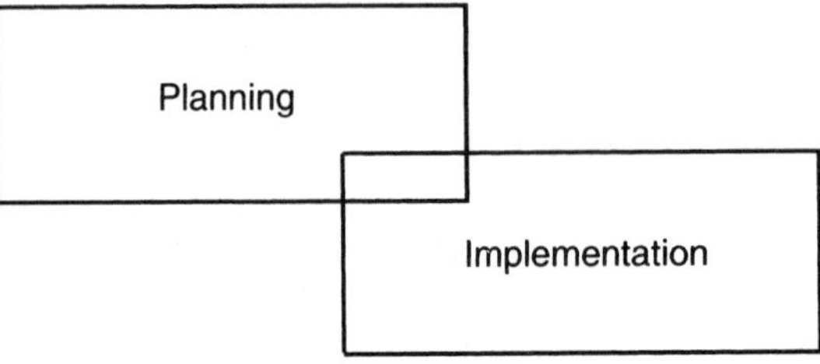

Implementation and Evaluation

Implementation and *Evaluation* overlap for an obvious reason: you don't blindly implement a plan of action without evaluating initial responses to your actions. Early in the implementation phase, you begin to evaluate whether the plan is working based on initial responses. You then make changes as needed before moving on to the formal evaluation phase.

The diagram below demonstrates the relationship between *Implementation* and *Evaluation.*

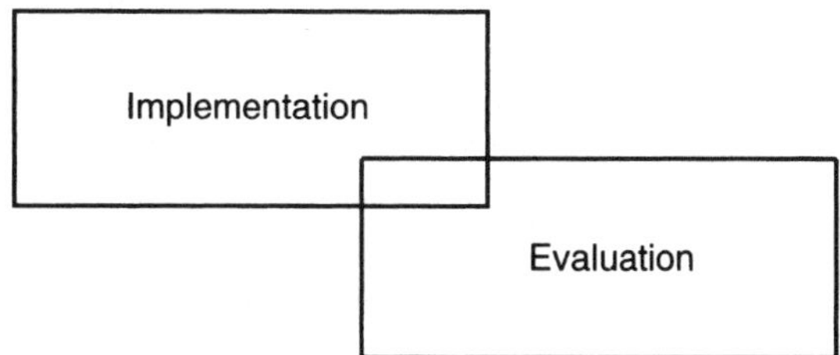
Implementation
Evaluation

Evaluation and the Other Steps in the Nursing Process

Evaluation is clearly related to *Planning* because, assuming your diagnoses are accurate and your outcomes are appropriate, the ultimate question to be answered during this phase is, "Have we achieved the outcomes determined during *Planning*?" However, because we can't just assume the diagnoses are accurate and outcomes appropriate, and because we need to identify things that helped or hindered progress, *Evaluation* involves examining *all of the other steps,* as illustrated below.

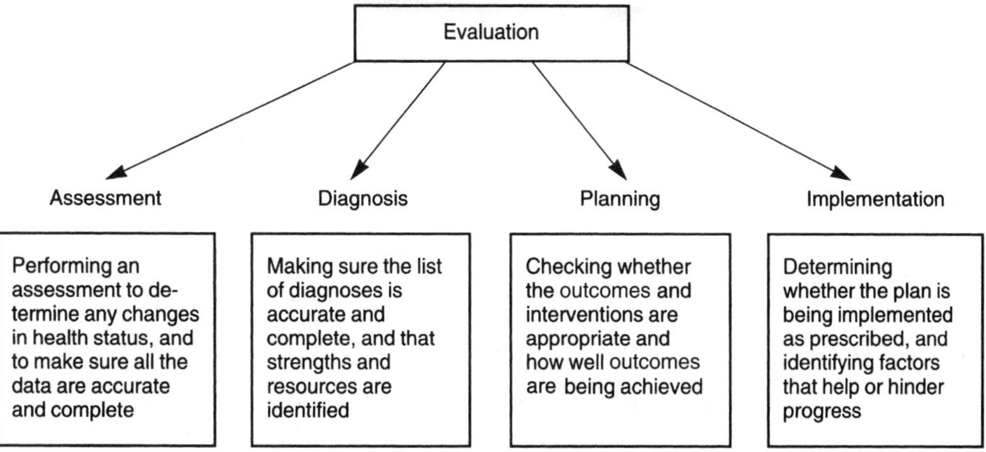
Evaluation
Assessment
Diagnosis
Planning
Implementation
Performing an assessment to determine any changes in health status, and to make sure all the data are accurate and complete
Making sure the list of diagnoses is accurate and complete, and that strengths and resources are identified
Checking whether the outcomes and interventions are appropriate and how well outcomes are being achieved
Determining whether the plan is being implemented as prescribed, and identifying factors that help or hinder progress

The following is an example of how the steps of the nursing process might be followed when caring for a specific person, Mr. Bagby.

- *Assessment:* Mr. Bagby complains his throat and mouth are dry. His temperature is elevated to 101°F. He's allowed fluids but has had almost nothing to drink all morning. He tells you he would push himself to drink, but he doesn't like water, especially when warm, and he hates bothering the nurses for ice.

- *Diagnosis:* You analyze the above data and identify *Fluid Volume Deficit related to insufficient fluid intake and fever*. You also recognize his willingness to increase fluids is a strength.
- *Planning:* Together with Mr. Bagby, you develop a plan of action by setting an expected outcome of maintaining adequate hydration by his drinking at least 2500 mL/day. You identify interventions to achieve the outcome and record the plan of care.
- *Implementation:* You ensure that favorite fluids are kept at the bedside on ice and monitor how Mr. Bagby is doing in meeting his daily goal.
- *Evaluation:* You assess Mr. Bagby and determine whether he still has *Fluid Volume Deficit*. If he is adequately hydrated and no longer at risk for *Fluid Volume Deficit* (ie, no longer has a fever), then you terminate the plan and allow him to follow his usual pattern of fluid intake. If he isn't adequately hydrated, you examine the steps above, identify factors that are inhibiting outcome achievement, and modify the plan accordingly.

Figure 1-1 summarizes the relationships among the steps of the nursing process.

What Are the Benefits of Using the Nursing Process?

The nursing process complements what other disciplines do by focusing on the *human response*—that is, how the person *responds to* medical problems, treatment plans, and

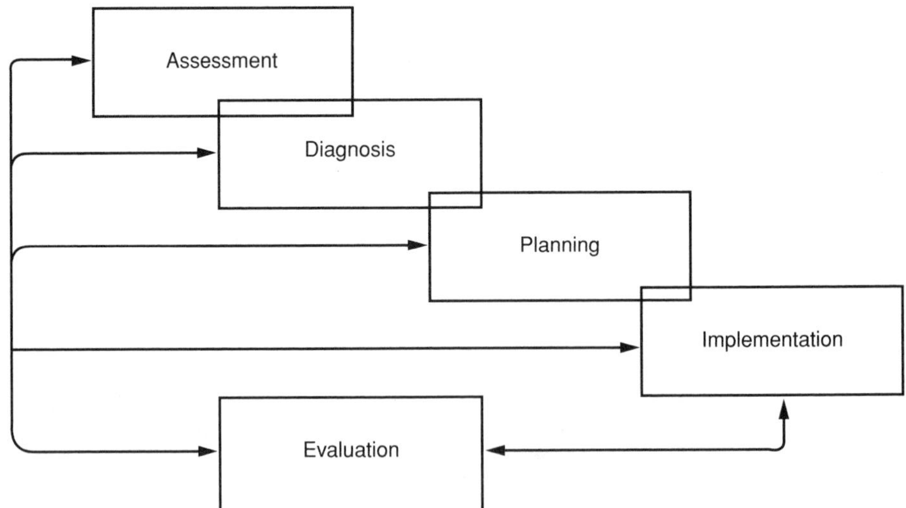

Figure **1–1.** Each step of the nursing process is dependent upon the accuracy of the preceding step. The steps are also overlapping because you may have to move quicker for some problems than others. *Evaluation* involves examining all the previous steps, but especially focuses on outcome achievement. The arrows between *Assessment* and *Evaluation* and between *Evaluation* and *Implementation* go in both directions because *Assessment* and *Evaluation* are *ongoing processes* as well as separate phases.

changes in activities of daily life. For example, if you had someone with a broken leg, you wouldn't only focus on treating the leg. You'd also be concerned with finding out about what having a broken leg *means to the person as a whole* (what problems does it cause to that specific individual).

This holistic focus helps ensure that interventions are tailored to the individual, not just the disease. Can you think what it would be like if you were hospitalized with a head laceration, a fractured arm, and a bruised kidney and everyone focused only on the medical problems? Can you imagine lying there with daily visits from a surgeon to check your head, an orthopedist to look at your arm, a urologist to check your kidney, and no one there to be concerned with how *you're* doing—to care about what *you* need and want?

There are other real, tangible benefits of using the nursing process, and these are summarized in Display 1-2. Display 1-3 compares how physicians and nurses may differ in their focus of assessment, diagnosis, and treatment of the same patient. Table 1-2 compares the nursing process and the medical process.

Ethics: Protecting Client Rights

A key part of your role as a nurse is that of being a client advocate. It's your responsibility to make sure that decisions and actions performed on behalf of clients are determined ethically. Before going on, take a few moments to review Display 1-4 (page 14), which addresses your responsibilities related to giving care in an ethical manner according to the American Nurses Association (ANA).

DISPLAY 1-2 Benefits of Using the Nursing Process

- Expedites diagnosis and treatment of actual and potential health problems, reducing the incidence of (and length of) hospital stays.
- Creates a plan that's cost-effective, both in terms of human suffering and monetary expense.
- Has precise documentation requirements designed to:
  - Improve communication, and to prevent errors, omissions, and unnecessary repetitions.
  - Leave a "paper trail" that can later be followed for evaluating patient care and for the purpose of doing studies that can advance nursing and improve the quality and efficiency of health care.
- Prevents clinicians from losing sight of the importance of the human factor.
- Promotes flexibility and independent thinking.
- Tailors interventions for the individual (not just the disease).
- Helps:
  - Patients and significant others realize their input is important and strong points are assets.
  - Nurses have the satisfaction of getting results.

DISPLAY 1-3 Example of How Nurses and Physicians Differ in Their Approaches to Assessment, Diagnosis, and Treatment

Physician's Data

Disease focus

"Mrs. Garcia has pain and swelling in all joints. Diagnostic studies indicate she has rheumatoid arthritis. We will start her on course of antiinflammatories to treat the rheumatoid arthritis."

(*Physician focuses on treating the arthritis.*)

Nurse's Data

Holistic focus, considering both problems and their effect on the patient/family

"Mrs. Garcia has pain and swelling in all joints, making it difficult to feed and dress herself. She has voiced that it's difficult to feel worthwhile when she can't even feed herself. She states she is depressed because she misses seeing her two small grandchildren. We need to develop a plan to help her with her pain, to assist her with feeding and dressing, to work through feelings of low self-esteem, and for special visitations with the grandchildren."

(*Nurse focuses on Mrs. Garcia's response* to arthritic changes and pain and how these impair everyday functioning as a biopsychosocial individual.)

TABLE 1–2 Comparison of Nursing Process and Medical Process

Nursing Process	Medical Process
Mainly considers how patients and families are affected by organ or system function (human responses).	Mainly considers organ and system function.
Focuses on teaching individuals or groups how to be independent in activities of daily living.	Focuses on teaching about how diseases and trauma are treated.
Consults with medicine for treatment of diseases or trauma.	Consults with nursing for planning for activities of daily life.
Involved with individuals, their significant others, and with groups.	Mostly involved with individuals, sometimes with groups and families.

Think About It

Carpenito (1997b) offers the following thought-provoking assumptions about the terms client, health, environment, *and* nursing:

Client: *Refers to an individual, group, or community; has the power for self-healing; continually interrelates with the environment; makes decisions according to*

individual priorities; is a unified whole, seeking balance; has individual worth and dignity; is an expert on own health.

Health: *Is dynamic, ever-changing state; is defined by the client; is an expression of optimum level of well-being; is the responsibility of the client.*

Environment: *Represents external factors, situations, and persons who influence or are influenced by the client; includes physical and ecologic environments, life events, and treatment modalities.*

Nursing: *Is accessed by the client when assistance is needed to improve, restore or maintain health or to achieve a peaceful death; engages the client to assume responsibility in self-healing decisions and practices; reduces or eliminates environmental factors that can or do cause compromised functioning.*

About the practice sessions throughout this book

The point of the practice sessions is to allow you to master content and practice critical thinking skills, not to make you do time-consuming writing exercises. You may either write your answers, explain them to someone else, verbalize them out loud to yourself, or tape record them. If you feel you don't need the practice, skip the session entirely. The answers provided in the back of the book are example responses*—they aren't the* only answers. *They are provided to allow you to evaluate and correct your own thinking. If you doubt whether your response is acceptable, ask your instructor.*

PRACTICE SESSION I

Steps of the Nursing Process

To complete this session, read pages 2–13. Example responses can be found on page 231.

1. Using terms a lay person can understand, explain:

   See pg 231

   a. The steps of the nursing process.

   Assessment
   Diagnosis
   Planning
   Implementation
   Evaluation

   b. Five advantages of using the nursing process.

   requirement set forth by national practice standards.
   provides basis for state board exam ques.
   promotes critical thinking in clinical setting

2. Give three reasons why you need to learn about nursing process.

3. The accuracy of the steps of the nursing process depends on the accuracy of the previous step (the accuracy of *Diagnosis* depends on the accuracy of *Assessment*, and so on). Explain why.

Try This on Your Own

The "Think About It" on page 12 has some powerful implications. Discuss each of the assumptions with one or more students, addressing whether you agree and what they imply for your work as a nurse.

Knowledge, Skills, and Caring: The Heart of Nursing Process Expertise

Now that you know what the nursing process is and why we use it, let's look at what it takes to be competent in its use. The diagram on p. 15 illustrates "the heart" of the nursing process: knowledge, skills, and caring. Notice that where knowledge (what to, why to), skills (how to), and caring (willing to, able to) come together is where you find nursing process expertise. Here's where the heart of the nursing process lies, where knowledge, skills, and caring come together as the driving force for quality care.

DISPLAY 1-4 Ethics: Protecting Client Rights*

As a nurse, you're responsible for:

- ✓ Following the *Code of Ethics* (ANA, 1985; see appendix, page 237).
- ✓ Maintaining client confidentiality.
- ✓ Acting as a client advocate.
- ✓ Seeking available resources to help formulate ethical decisions.
- ✓ Delivering care in a way that is
  - nonjudgmental, nondiscriminatory, and sensitive to client diversity
  - preserves and protects client autonomy, dignity, and rights.

*From: American Nurses Association. *Standards of Clinical Nursing Practice: Standards of Professional Performance (1991)*. Washington, DC ANA.

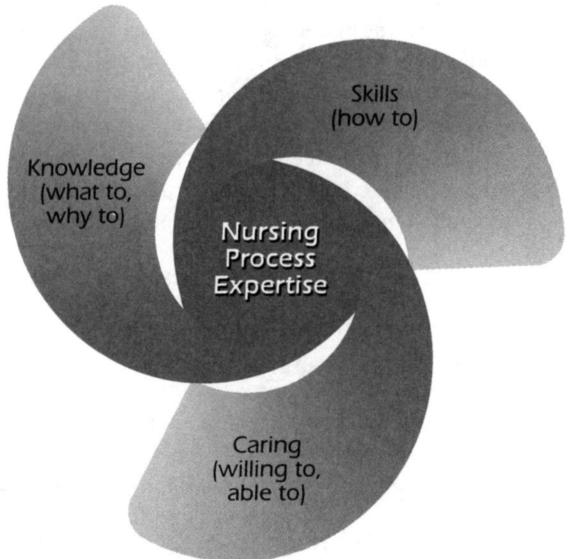

You may look at the above illustration and feel that you're limited in one area or another (eg, your knowledge is stronger than your skills). In fact, most nurses feel stronger in one area than another. Keeping this illustration in mind and recognizing areas that need development can help you set realistic expectations for yourself. It will also help you identify ways to improve. As you complete this section and the following chapters, studying each step of the nursing process in more depth, you'll see that you'll get closer and closer to seeing yourself in the section labeled nursing process expertise. You'll gain knowledge about what to and why to, you'll practice the skills of how to, and you'll identify what it takes to be willing and able to care.

Nursing Knowledge: Broad and Varied

The knowledge base that guides nursing actions is broad and varied, including all of the following:

- Health promotion
- Growth and development
- Mental health/psychiatry
- Community health/group dynamics
- Cultures/ethics/law
- Research/leadership
- Teaching/counseling
- Communication/negotiation
- Problem solving/critical thinking
- Computers/Technology
- Anatomy and physiology
- Nursing diagnosis/nursing process
- Nursing care management
- Disease process/treatment
- Diagnostic/monitoring modalities
- Pathophysiology/pharmacology
- Microbiology/chemistry
- Physical and social sciences
- Practice wisdom*

* Practice wisdom includes experiential knowledge (eg, what abnormal breathsounds sound like) and knowledge of tradition, ethics, authority, trial and error, intuition, and rules of logic.

If you're a beginning student, your nursing knowledge is limited. You might feel like you're struggling to use the nursing process. You know the steps but need to know more about the problems and approaches to solving the problems. However, as you continue your education and increase your knowledge of the above areas, you'll become more proficient. If you internalize the principles and rules on which the nursing process is based, making them habits of performance early on, you'll be able to make the most of your limited knowledge. You may not know everything, but you'll know what resources to use, where to go for information, and how to act safely.

Skills: Manual, Intellectual, Interpersonal

Using the nursing process effectively requires manual, intellectual, and interpersonal skills. You need manual skills to complete technical procedures, intellectual skills to solve problems and make decisions, and interpersonal skills to establish good interpersonal relationships with patients, significant others, and coworkers. Skills labs and clinical experiences provide the opportunity for developing manual skills; this section addresses how to develop intellectual and interpersonal skills.

Intellectual Skills: Critical Thinking

Unlike the almost mindless thinking we do when going about our daily routine, critical thinking is careful, deliberate, goal-directed thinking. Display 1-5 defines critical thinking in nursing and gives examples of when it's essential to use critical thinking.

How to Become a Critical Thinker

Most people learn critical thinking in two phases: First you learn general critical thinking skills for everyday situations, then you learn more specific skills that require specific knowledge. For example, in lower grades, you learn general problem-solving principles that can be applied to everyday situations. Now, as a nurse, you need to acquire nursing knowledge and experience to be able to develop problem-solving skills specific to nursing.

In one way, critical thinking is like any other skill: If you practice it, it becomes more automatic. The exercises throughout this book are intended to help you develop, refine, and practice your ability to think critically in the context of nursing situations. As you complete each chapter, learning and applying the principles and rules that guide you to use the nursing process, you'll begin to develop habits that will help you be more automatic in your approaches to nursing situations. For now, take a few moments to look at Display 1-6 (p. 18), which lists some characteristics of critical thinkers, and evaluate your current habits of thinking. Check each characteristic and ask yourself, "Is this me?" Put a mark next to the ones you want to develop or improve.

Interpersonal Skills

Developing interpersonal skills is as important as developing critical thinking skills. If you're unable to establish positive interpersonal relationships, you're unlikely to get the real facts, understand the real problems, get others to help, or be an effective member of the health care team.

DISPLAY 1-5 What Is Critical Thinking in Nursing?*

Critical Thinking in Nursing:

- Entails purposeful, goal-directed thinking.
- Aims to make judgments based on evidence (fact), rather than conjecture (guesswork).
- Is based on principles of science and the scientific method (eg, maintaining a questioning attitude, following an organized approach to discovery, and making sure information is reliable).
- Is constantly reevaluating, self-correcting, and striving to improve.
- Requires knowledge, skills, and experience.
- Requires strategies that maximize *human potential* (using individual strengths) and compensate for problems created by *human nature* (eg, the powerful influence of personal perceptions, values, and beliefs).

Examples of When Critical Thinking is Essential:

When trying to:

- Get a better understanding of someone or something
- Identify actual and potential problems
- Make decisions about an action plan
- Reduce risks of getting undesirable results
- Increase the likelihood of achieving beneficial results
- Find ways to improve (even when no problem exists)

*Adapted from: Alfaro-LeFevre, 1996.

Many believe that communication skills are the key to positive interpersonal relationships. However, good communication skills are really only half of what's required to build sound interpersonal relationships. Relationships are developed as much by how we *behave* as by how we communicate—actions speak louder than words. To establish positive interpersonal relationships, you must develop behaviors that send messages like, I'm reliable . . . , I respect you . . . , You can trust me . . . , and I want to do a good job.

Although I don't intend to diminish the value of communication skills, I'll wait to discuss these in the next chapter, when we discuss and practice communication techniques in the section on interviewing. For now, think about the messages sent by behavior. Look at Table 1-3 (p. 20), which describes behaviors that enhance interpersonal relationships and those that inhibit interpersonal relationships. Consider some behaviors you'd like to develop or improve.

Willingness and Ability to Care

We've discussed the importance of knowledge and skills. Now let's look at the third component of nursing process expertise, *caring*.

DISPLAY 1-6 Characteristics of Critical Thinkers

Critical Thinkers Are:

- **Aware of their strengths and capabilities:** They're confident that they can reason to find answers and make good decisions.
- **Sensitive to their own limitations and predispositions:** They know their weaknesses, values, and beliefs and recognize when these may hamper their ability to assess a situation or solve a problem.
- **Open minded:** They listen to new ideas and viewpoints and consider the situation from many perspectives.
- **Humble:** They overcome their own tendency to feel that they should have all the answers.
- **Creative:** They are constantly looking for better ways to get things done. They follow recommended procedures, however, they continually examine whether these are the best ways to meet goals and objectives.
- **Proactive:** They accept responsibility and accountability for their actions. They study situations, anticipate problems, and find ways to avoid them *before* they happen.
- **Flexible:** They recognize the importance of changing priorities and interventions when planned approaches don't seem to be getting results.
- **Aware that errors are stepping stones to new ideas:** They turn mistakes into learning opportunities, reflecting on what went wrong and identifying ways to avoid the same mistake in the future.
- **Willing to persevere:** They know that sometimes there are no easy answers and that there may be time-consuming struggles to find the best answer.
- **Cognizant of the fact that we don't live in a perfect world:** They realize that sometimes the *best* answer may not be the *perfect* answer.
- **Introspective:** They evaluate and correct their own thinking.

Critical Thinkers Also:

- **Maintain a questioning attitude:** They ask questions like, "What's going on here?"; "What does it mean?"; and "What else could it mean, and how else could it be interpreted?"
- **Ask for clarification when they don't understand:** For example, they say, "I'm not clear about this. Can you tell me more?" *or* ask questions like, "What do you mean by *better*, better in what way?"
- **Apply previous knowledge to new situations**: They see similarities and differences between one experience and another, between one concept and another.
- **See the situation from many perspectives:** They value all viewpoints and watch that their judgments are based on *facts*, not personal feelings, views, or self-interest.
- **Weigh risks and benefits (advantages and disadvantages) before making a decision:** They avoid risky decisions and find ways to reduce adverse reactions before putting a plan into action.
- **Seek help when needed.**
- **Put first things first:** They ask, "What's the most important thing to do here?"

(continued)

DISPLAY 1-6 Characteristics of Critical Thinkers (Continued)

Critical Thinkers Use Logic. They:

- **Test first impressions to make sure they are as they appear:** They double check the logic of their thinking and the workability of their solutions.
- **Distinguish between fact and fallacy:** They take the time to verify important information to be sure it's true.
- **Distinguish fact from inference (what they *believe* the fact means):** For example, they recognize that because someone is sitting quietly in a corner may not mean that the individual is *withdrawn*; it means that they are sitting quietly in a corner and that it would be helpful to find out why.
- **Support views with evidence:** They wouldn't state that the person above is withdrawn without providing additional supporting evidence, such as the individual saying he wants nothing to do with anyone.
- **Determine what's relevant and what's irrelevant:** They recognize what's important for understanding a situation and what's unimportant. For example, the fact that you're a nurse or studying to be a nurse is relevant to how I should write this book; the fact that you are female or male is irrelevant.
- **Apply the concept of "cause and effect":** They look for what's causing a problem to more fully understand the problem itself. They anticipate responses to their actions before performing the action. For example, critical thinkers would attempt to find out the *cause* of pain before deciding how to *treat* it. They would determine how someone might *respond* to a medication before *administering* it.
- **Withhold judgment until all the necessary facts are in:** They realize the dangers of jumping to conclusions.

Willingness to Care

Being willing to care means making the choice to do what it takes to help others. This includes choosing to

- Keep the focus on what's best for the consumer (person, family, community).
- Respect the values and beliefs of others.
- Stay involved, even when problems become chronic or more severe.
- Maintain a healthy lifestyle so you're able to help.

In addition to the above, the ANA addresses standards of professional performance, or professional behaviors that enhance use of the nursing process (See Display 1-7, p. 21). Being willing to care involves being willing to work toward making these behaviors habits of performance. The case study on page 21 demonstrates how applying some of these behaviors can make a significant difference in the quality of patient care and job satisfaction.

TABLE 1–3 Behaviors Affecting Interpersonal Relationships

Behaviors That Enhance Interpersonal Relationships	Behaviors That Inhibit Interpersonal Relationships
Conveying an attitude of openness, acceptance, and lack of prejudice.	Conveying an attitude of doubt, mistrust, or negative judgment.
Being honest.	Giving false information.
Taking initiative and responsibility; responding to others' concerns.	Conveying an "it's not my job" attitude.
Being reliable.	Not meeting commitments, only partially meeting commitments, or not being punctual.
Demonstrating humility.	Demonstrating self-importance.
Showing respect for what others are, have been, or may become.	"Talking down" or assuming familiarity.
Accepting accountability.	Making excuses or placing blame where it doesn't belong.
Being confident and prepared.	Being unsure and trying to "wing it."
Showing genuine interest.	Acting like you're only doing something because it's a job.
Conveying appreciation for others' time.	Assuming others have more time than we do.
Accepting expression of positive *and* negative feelings.	Demonstrating discomfort when negative feelings are expressed.
Taking enough time.	Rushing.
Being frank and forthright.	Sending mixed messages, saying things just because we think it's what the other person seems to want to hear, or talking behind others' backs.
Admitting when we've been wrong.	Denying or ignoring when we've made an error.
Apologizing if we've caused distress or inconvenience.	Acting like nothing happened or making excuses.
Being willing to forgive and forget.	Holding grudges.
Showing a positive attitude.	Conveying an "it'll never work" attitude.
Conveying a sense of humor.	Acting like there's no room for anything but "serious business."
Allowing others control.	Trying to control others.
Giving credit where credit is due.	Ignoring achievements or taking credit that doesn't belong to us.

DISPLAY 1-7 ANA Standards of Professional Performance* (Professional Behavior)

Standard I **Quality of Care**: The nurse systematically evaluates the quality and effectiveness of nursing practice.

II **Performance Appraisal:** The nurse evaluates his/her own nursing practice in relation to professional practice standards and relevant statutes and regulations.

III **Education:** The nurse acquires and maintains current knowledge in nursing practice.

IV **Collegiality:** The nurse contributes to the professional development of peers, colleagues, and others.

V **Ethics:** The nurse's decisions and actions on behalf of clients are determined in an ethical manner.

VI **Collaboration:** The nurse collaborates with the client, significant others, and health care providers in providing client care.

VII **Research:** The nurse uses research findings in practice.

VIII **Resource Utilization:** The nurse considers factors related to safety, effectiveness, and cost in planning and delivering client care.

*From: *Standards of Clinical Practice* (1991). American Nurses Association. Washington, DC.

CASE STUDY

How Using Resources, Applying Research, and Using a Collegial Approach to Collaborate Can Make a Difference in Care Quality and Job Satisfaction

Mr. Moran has chronic lung disease and has been on nasal oxygen at home for the past 6 months. He's been admitted for evaluation of possible heart problems. Bruce Franklin is Mr. Moran's nurse. Dr. Kenny is his physician. Bruce notes that Mr. Moran continues to have extreme difficulty breathing any time he moves around, even with his oxygen on. Although Dr. Kenny is aware of this, she's had some other major priorities and hasn't been able to focus on Mr. Moran's chronic breathing problems.

Bruce begins to wonder if something could be done to improve the situation. He asks Dee Baker, the respiratory clinical nurse specialist, if she would discuss Mr. Moran's care with him. They set aside time to discuss Mr. Moran's care. Dee mentions she's read about the benefits of transtracheal oxygen delivery. She asks the librarian to do a computer search on transtracheal oxygen delivery, and two research articles are found. Dee and Bruce review the articles and learn that transtracheal oxygen delivery may be more effective than nasal cannula oxygen delivery. Bruce asks for a copy of the research articles for his files.

Bruce and the clinical specialist discuss the findings with Dr. Kenny, resulting in new orders of transtracheal oxygen delivery. Mr. Moran demonstrates a significant improvement in ability to tolerate activity. Bruce has the satisfaction of knowing he made a difference and gained knowledge of treatment modalities. Dee has the satisfaction of knowing she's made a difference in two lives, Mr. Moran's and Bruce's. The next time she sees the librarian, she lets her know that her computer search benefited all involved. Dr. Kenny is pleased to know that she has two dependable colleagues who are independent thinkers, use resources, and are willing to work as a team to make a difference. ■

Display 1-8 lists some behaviors you can use to show patients and families you care.

Being Able to Care

Being able to care requires understanding ourselves and understanding others.

Understanding Ourselves

Learning to understand ourselves is a lifelong pursuit. Gaining insight into ourselves involves learning about our tendencies, reactions, and habits, and these tend to change as we grow and mature. By making a commitment to learn about ourselves and recognize how our values and frame of reference might influence our thinking and ability to understand others, we can take deliberate steps to be more objective in our thinking.

Understanding Others

Understanding others takes learning how to listen empathetically, or to listen with the intent to enter into another's way of thinking and viewing the world (Covey, 1989). Some use the analogy of trying to view the world through someone else's glasses or trying to walk in another's shoes. (Both are often almost impossible!) Listening empathet-

DISPLAY 1-8 Ten Caring Behaviors

1. Inspiring someone, or instilling hope and faith (creating a vision of what is or could be).
2. Demonstrating patience, compassion, and willingness to persevere.
3. Offering companionship (eg, listening, or being with someone for no other reason than to listen or *be* with the person).
4. Helping someone stay in touch with positive aspects of his life (eg, inquiring about significant others, pets, special interests, or hobbies).
5. Demonstrating thoughtfulness (eg, calling or visiting someone for no other reason than knowing it will let the person know you're thinking of him).
6. Bending the rules when it really counts (eg, arranging for a pet to visit).
7. Doing the "little things" and the "extra things."
8. Taking the time required, rather than hurrying through just to get things done.
9. Keeping someone informed.
10. Showing your human side by sharing "stories" (exchanging tales of special interests and activities).

ically takes letting go of how we, ourselves, view the world and connecting with another's feelings and perceptions. It takes identifying with another's struggles, frustrations, and desires. And then it takes detaching from the feelings, and returning to our own frame of reference. Once we've detached, we're likely to be more objective and still be able to understand what's important to the person. We'll be more able to identify needs, prioritize problems, and find common goals. Display 1-9 on p. 24 provides steps for listening empathetically.

The following case study demonstrates how these steps might be used in a real situation.

CASE STUDY

Example of How Listening Empathetically Promotes Understanding of the Real Issues and Fosters Caring for Human Responses

Today Pat is caring for Sharon, who's just given birth to her fifth child, a healthy baby girl. Pat has never been able to conceive, has always wanted children, and feels a little envious of Sharon's family of two boys and (now) three girls.

Pat notes that Sharon seems very quiet. Recognizing the importance of being an empathetic listener, Pat has the following conversation with Sharon. ■

Pat: "You've been pretty quiet since I came on."

Sharon: "I can't help it. I'm supposed to be happy, but I'm really disappointed—I was so sure I'd have a boy."

Pat (making a conscious effort to eliminate thoughts about the fact that she'd be happy with any child, and rephrasing what Sharon seems to be feeling): "You feel like you're supposed to be happy, but you really feel sort of sad?"

Sharon: "Yes."
Pat pauses to reflect on the feeling of sadness and encourage Sharon to continue.

Sharon: "I was going to name this baby after my father. He died 2 months ago."

Pat (connecting to what Sharon must be feeling): "I'm sorry. That would be a disappointment. Being able to name the baby after him would have been a lovely thing to do."

Sharon (crying): "Yes. I had it all pictured in my mind."

Pat, conveying acceptance and understanding, sits quietly, allowing Sharon to cry.

Pat (detaching and coming back to her own frame of reference): "Sharon, I think you needed to cry, and you may need to cry again. But right now you've got a beautiful baby girl with the longest hair I've ever seen waiting to meet her mother. How would you feel if I brought her in to you?"

Sharon: "Yes. I really haven't seen her for more than 5 minutes (smiling). It's not her fault she's a girl. I've got to admit, I've always gotten along better with my girls than my boys."

DISPLAY 1-9 Steps for Listening Empathetically

1. Eliminate thoughts about how *you* see the other person's situation.
2. Listen carefully for *feelings* and try to identify with how the *other person* perceives his situation. Don't allow yourself to think about how you're going to respond; think only about the *content* of what you're hearing.
3. Reflect on what you've been told, then rephrase the *feelings*.
4. Seek validation that you've understood the message, content, and emotion correctly. Keep trying until you're sure you understand.
5. Detach, and come back to your own frame of reference.

PRACTICE SESSION II

Critical Thinking, Interpersonal Skills, and Willingness and Ability to Care

To complete this session, read pages14–24. Unless an asterisk is placed after the number, an example response to each question can be found on page 231.

1. List five critical thinking characteristics you'd like to acquire or improve.

2. Complete the following sentence, using as many words as you choose: *If I were to tell someone how I think, I would say that I . . .* (No example response given).

3. What does critical thinking in nursing mean to you?

4. Give three examples of caring behaviors.

patience Keeping someone
Companionship informed

5. Study Display 1–10 (*Nursing's Social Policy Statement*, 1995). Choose one statement and explain what it means to you. (No example response given).

Try This on Your Own

1. **Gain Insight Into Interpersonal Skills:** In a group, or with a friend, think of some examples that demonstrate each of the behaviors listed in Table 1–3 that enhance or inhibit interpersonal relationships.
2. **Gain Insight Into Yourself:** With a friend, or in a group, discuss some of your tendencies, behaviors, attitudes, and reactions. Discuss how you are similar to others and how you're different. Identify some behaviors in others that are difficult for you to accept. Explain how you react when you encounter these behaviors. Think of ways you could change.

   In the case history on page 21, everyone works well together and is happy with the results. However, in the real world, one or two of the people involved may come away with bruised feelings. Who might these people be? What, If anything, could be done about it?

   Review the case history on page 23. Consider what might have happened if Sharon hadn't deliberately used the steps of *empathetic listening*.
3. **Practice Empathetic Listening.** Ask someone to tell you about an upsetting experience in his childhood, and listen using the steps of empathetic listening listed in Display 1–9.

DISPLAY 1–10 Nursing's Social Policy Statement (1995)*

Statements on the Importance of Caring, and Cultural and Spiritual Factors

- An essential feature of contemporary nursing practice is the provision of a caring relationship that facilitates healing (p. 6).
- Humans manifest an essential unity of mind/body/spirit (p. 3).
- Human experience is contextually and culturally defined (p. 3).

Other Key Statements Related to This Chapter

- Health and illness are human experiences (p. 4).
- The presence of illness does not preclude health nor does optimal health preclude illness (p. 4).

*Adapted from Alfaro-LeFevre workshop handouts © 1995.

Summary

The nursing process is required by national practice standards, provides the basis for state board exam questions, and helps you think critically in the clinical setting. Its five steps—*Assessment, Diagnosis, Planning, Implementation, Evaluation*—

overlap and are interrelated. The accuracy of each step depends on the accuracy of the preceding step. Using the nursing process complements what other disciplines (physicians, physical therapists, and so forth) do by focusing on the *human response*—that is, how the person *responds to* medical problems, treatment plans, and changes in activities of daily life. Being competent in using the nursing process requires a combination of knowledge (what to, why to), skills (how to) and caring (willing to, able to). It requires a broad nursing knowledge base, clinical expertise and strong interpersonal skills.

Evaluate your knowledge of this chapter. Check to see if you can achieve the objectives on page 189.

Bibliography: See page 191.

CHAPTER 2

Assessment

OBJECTIVES

Once you complete this chapter, you should be able to:

- Describe five phases of *Assessment.*
- Explain why having incomplete or incorrect assessment data affects the entire plan of care.
- Compare and contrast the terms *data base assessment* and *focus assessment.*
- Discuss ethical, cultural, and spiritual considerations related to performing an assessment.
- Explain how the interview and physical assessment complement and clarify each other.
- Give an example of an open-ended question, closed-ended question, leading question, and exploratory statement.
- Describe how you plan to perform an interview and physical examination the next time you're in the clinical setting.
- Identify subjective and objective data in a nursing assessment.
- Differentiate between cues and inferences.
- Explain why organizing data according to more than one method (eg, body systems and a nursing model) promotes critical thinking.
- Give a detailed account of how you'll perform a comprehensive assessment the next time you're in the clinical setting.
- Explain how you'll decide what information to report and record the next time you're in the clinical setting.

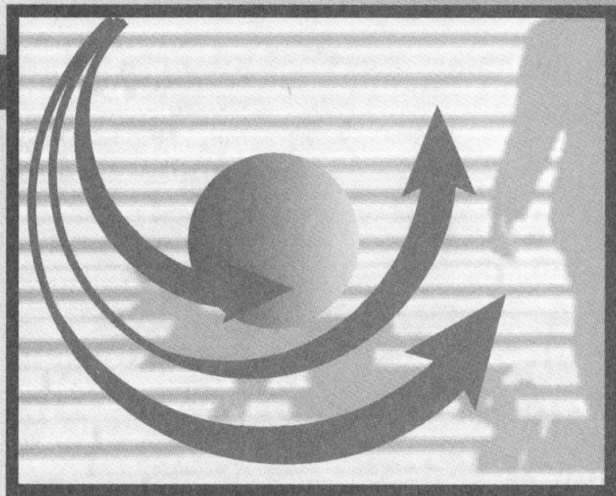

Standard I. ***Assessment.*** The nurse collects client health data.*

Practice Sessions

- **Practice Session III:** The Nursing Interview and Physical Assessment
- **Practice Session IV:** Subjective and Objective Data; Cues and Inferences; Validating Data
- **Practice Session V:** Organizing (Clustering) Data
- **Practice Session VI:** Recognizing Abnormal Data, Deciding What's Relevant, Applying the Principle of Cause and Effect

What's in this chapter?

Emphasizing the point that the entire plan of care depends on the accuracy and completeness of *Assessment,* this chapter examines how to assess in a way that facilitates the next step, *Diagnosis.* It explains the *how to's* and the *why's* of the five key activities of *Assessment* (collecting data, validating data, clustering data, identifying patterns/testing first impressions, and reporting and recording data).

*Excerpted from ANA Standards of Clinical Nursing Practice (ANA, 1991).

Assessment: The First Step to Determining Health Status

Assessment is the first step to determining health status. It's when you gather information to make sure you have all the "necessary puzzle pieces" to put together a clear picture of the person's health state. Because the entire plan of care is based on the data you collect during this phase, make every effort to ensure that your information is correct, complete, and organized in a way that you'll begin to get a sense of patterns of health or illness.

There are five key activities that can help you perform the systematic, comprehensive assessment that's so crucial to recognizing and treating health problems in a safe and timely fashion.

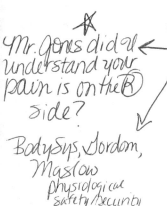

- *Collecting Data:* You gather health status data.
- *Validating (Verifying) Data:* You validate that your data is accurate and complete.
- *Organizing Data:* You cluster the data into groups of information that help you identify patterns of health or illness (eg, you cluster all data about nutrition together, all the data about activity together, and so forth).
- *Identifying Patterns/Testing First Impressions:* You get an initial idea of patterns of function, and focus your assessment to gain more information to better understand the situation at hand. For example, you may begin to think someone seems to have a pattern of poor nutrition and decide to find out what's contributing to this pattern (does the person have poor eating habits or could it be something else, like lack of available refrigeration?).
- *Reporting and Recording Data:* You report significant data (eg, a high fever) and complete the patient's record. Reporting significant data before you chart ensures that other responsible members of the health care team are immediately aware of your major concerns.

Collecting Data

Collecting data is an ongoing process. It begins when you first meet the patient, and it continues with each subsequent encounter until the person is discharged. Let's take a look at the resources and methods you use to gather information about someone's health status.

What Resources Do You Use to Gather Data?

The bullets below summarize the resources to consider to ensure comprehensive assessment. However, remember that your direct examination and interview of the person requiring care are likely to provide the most significant information.

- Consumer (person, family, community)
- Significant others
- Nursing records
- Medical records
- Verbal and written consultations
- Diagnostic studies
- Relevant literature

Some facilities classify data into two categories: direct and indirect data. *Direct data* is information you gained directly from the person requiring care (eg, from your interview and examination). *Indirect data* is information gained from other sources (eg, a spouse, another nurse).

How Can You Ensure Comprehensive Data Collection?

Comprehensive data collection usually occurs in three phases:

1. **Before you see the person:** You find out what you can. This information may be very limited (only name and age), or quite extensive (you may be able to read medical records).
2. **When you see the person:** You perform an interview and physical examination.
3. **After you see the person:** You review the resources you've used and determine what other resources may offer additional information (eg, you may talk with a social worker or consult with a pharmacist to gain more information about a medication regimen).

Data Base Assessment and Focus Assessment

There are two main types of assessment:

- Data Base Assessment: Comprehensive information you gather on initial contact with the person to assess *all aspects* of health status.
- Focus Assessment: The data you gather to determine the status of a *specific condition* (eg, someone's bowel habits).

Data Base Assessment

Because of the importance of comprehensive data collection, virtually all facilities have standardized their assessment tools, also called data base forms. There are three major factors that may influence how these tools are designed and what information is required:

1. The needs and problems commonly encountered on the specific unit. For example, an assessment tool for an adult is different from an assessment tool for an infant (Figure 2–1, page 32) and an assessment tool for acute care is different from one for a long-term care facility (compare Figures 2–2, page 33, and 2–3, page 37).
2. The nursing model or theory adopted by facility (Functional Health Patterns, Self-Care Theory, Human Responses, and so forth).
3. Government, accrediting agency, professional standards, and insurance requirements. Some state and local governments require that certain information is recorded in a standard way (Display 2–1, p. 41). Agencies like The Joint Commission on Accreditation of Healthcare Organizations (JCAHO) and the Community Health Accreditation Program (CHAP) have published specific standards (JCAHO, 1994; CHAP, 1993). The ANA and other professional organizations, such as the American Associ-

ADULT ASSESSMENT TOOL: HEALTH PERCEPTION–HEALTH MAINTENANCE

Past History

Previous illnesses/hospitalizations
History of smoking/alcohol intake?
Exercise tolerance?
Patient's statement of past health status?
Medications?

INFANT ASSESSMENT TOOL: HEALTH PERCEPTION–HEALTH MAINTENANCE

Birth History

Prenatal:	Planned pregnancy? Weight gain? Complications?	Emotional response? Alcohol/Drug use?
Labor:	Length? Vaginal/Cesarean? Complications?	Spontaneous delivery? Anesthesia?
Bonding:	Major care giver?	Other family members?

Figure **2–1.** Excerpts from an adult assessment tool and an infant assessment tool showing how tools are tailor-made to meet the needs of specific populations.

ation of Critical Care Nurses (AACN), also publish specific standards. Insurance companies require specific information to verify the need for skilled nursing care.

How an assessment tool is organized and what information is gained by completing it influences your ability to collect relevant data. Having a holistic tool that's tailor-made to gain specific information about commonly encountered problems can be the key to getting pertinent, complete data. If you aren't familiar with the assessment tools your school or facility uses, make yourself a note now to request copies. You can then apply what you're reading in this chapter to what you'll actually be doing in the clinical area.

(text continued on page 41)

Think About It

Acquiring a well-designed assessment tool, then determining exactly why *every piece of information it guides you to collect is required helps you learn the critical thinking skill of* recognizing what's relevant *(eg, a maternity nursing assessment tool helps you learn what's relevant to the care of someone in labor).*

THE BRYN MAWR HOSPITAL
NURSING DEPARTMENT

NURSING ADMISSION ASSESSMENT

DATE 1/25/98 TIME OF ARRIVAL 8:00 AM

FROM ER

ACCOMPANIED BY Wife

VIA: WHEELCHAIR ✓ STRETCHER ___ AMBULATORY ___

ID BRACELET ✓ INFORMATION OBTAINED FROM Patient

I. VITAL STATISTICS

TEMP 101 PULSE 120 RESP 28

ORAL ✓ RECTAL ___ AXILLARY ___

BP RA 130/80 LA 128/80 POSITION Sitting

WEIGHT 158# HEIGHT 5'11"

SCALE: BED ___ CHAIR ___ STANDING ✓

DEFERRED ___

ORIENTED TO ROOM ✓

PROSTHESIS, APPLIANCES OR OTHER DEVICES

DENTURES 0 *WALKER/CANE/CRUTCHES 0

FULL: UPPER 0 LOWER 0 *ARTIFICIAL LIMBS 0

PARTIAL: UPPER 0 LOWER 0 *BRACES 0

EYE GLASSES ✓ *FALSE EYE 0

CONTACT LENSES 0 WIG 0

HEARING AID 0

OTHER 0

COMMENTS wearing glasses

PATIENT HAS BROUGHT TO HOSPITAL? YES ✓ NO ___

EXCEPTIONS ___

II. ALLERGIES: DRUGS 0 DYES 0 FOOD 0 OTHER ___ NONE KNOWN ✓

SPECIFY AGENT	DESCRIBE REACTION (IF KNOWN)
None	

III. HEALTH PERCEPTION–HEALTH MAINTENANCE

A. PRESENT ILLNESS

1. ADMITTING DIAGNOSIS UTI
2. REASON FOR ADMISSION (PATIENT STATEMENT) I think I have a urinary infection.
3. DURATION OF PRESENT ILLNESS 6 days
4. PAST AND PRESENT TREATMENT OF PRESENT ILLNESS AND RESPONSE Cipro X 7 days → cure
5. PATIENT AWARE OF DIAGNOSIS YES ✓ NO ___ NOT ESTABLISHED ___

B. PREVIOUS ILLNESSES (INCLUDING HOSPITALIZATION) 1990 Arrhythmia p̄ running. No MI.

Figure 2–2. Acute care assessment tool. (Adapted with permission from Bryn Mawr Hospital, Bryn Mawr, PA.)

C. ARE YOU TAKING ANY MEDICATIONS (PRESCRIBED OR OVER THE COUNTER) YES ✓ NO ___

MEDICATION	DOSE	WHEN DO YOU TAKE IT	WHY DO YOU TAKE IT	LAST DOSE	BROUGHT TO HOSPITAL YES	BROUGHT TO HOSPITAL NO	DISPOSITION
ASA	ii	PRN	Fever/Headache	6 A		✓	
Mylanta	ii tabs	PRN	Heartburn	days ago		✓	

D. DO YOU OR HAVE YOU EVER USED?

	YES	NO	LAST USED	FREQUENCY/AMOUNT
ALCOHOL	✓			
RECREATIONAL DRUGS				

E. DO YOU SMOKE? YES ___ PKS DAY ___ HOW LONG ___
(NO) DID YOU EVER SMOKE? NO ___ YES ✓ PKS DAY 1 HOW LONG 15yrs WHEN DID YOU QUIT 10 yrs.

IV. COGNITIVE PERCEPTUAL: HEADACHE ✓ SEIZURES 0 BLACKOUTS 0 DIZZINESS 0 NO C/O 0

A. LEVEL OF CONSCIOUSNESS: ALERT ✓ DROWSY ___ RESPONDS TO PAIN ___ VERBAL STIMULI ___ UNRESPONSIVE ___

B. ORIENTED TIME ✓ PLACE ✓ PERSON ✓ COMMENTS 0

C. MOOD RELAXED – ANXIOUS ✓ SAD – ANGRY – WITHDRAWN – OTHER –

D. RECENT MEMORY CHANGE YES ___ NO ✓ SPECIFY ___

E. RESPONDS TO DIRECTIONS YES ✓ NO ___ SPECIFY ___

F. SPEECH CLEAR ✓ SLURRED ___ GARBLED ___ UNABLE TO SPEAK ___ APHASIC ___

G. LANGUAGE SPOKEN ENGLISH ✓ OTHER ___

H. HEARING WNL ✓ IMPAIRED ___ CORRECTED ___ DEAF ___ SIGN LANGUAGE ___ LIP READS ___

I. VISION WNL ✓ IMPAIRED ___ CORRECTED ___ BLIND ___

J. PAIN YES ✓ NO ___ DESCRIBE Aches all over

HOW DO YOU MANAGE YOUR PAIN? ASA

K. LEARNING READINESS NO LIMITATIONS ✓ WILLING TO LEARN ___ RESISTS LEARNING ___

EMOTIONALLY READY TO LEARN YES ✓ NO ___ REQUIRES CONCRETE LANGUAGE REINFORCEMENT ___ FORGETFUL ___

TEACHING TO BE DIRECTED PRIMARILY TO patient

FAMILY MEMBER SIGNIFICANT OTHER

L. COMMENTS Knowledgeable about UTI

V. ROLE RELATIONSHIP (PSYCHOSOCIAL)/DISCHARGE PLANNING

A. OCCUPATION Salesman

B. LIVE ALONE ___ WITH FAMILY ✓ NURSING HOME ___ OTHER ___ COMMENT 2 children (8+10)

C. DESCRIBE PHYSICAL ENVIRONMENT Split level

D. ANTICIPATED DISCHARGE TO ECF No HOME CARE SERVICES 0

OTHER ___ HOME ___ IF GOING HOME, WHO COULD HELP YOU WITH

HEALTHCARE NEEDS AFTER DISCHARGE? Self-care

E. DO YOU WISH TO SEE A MEMBER OF THE CLERGY WHILE YOU ARE HERE? YES ___ NO ✓ AFFILIATION ___

F. COMMENTS 0

VI. HEALTH HISTORY ASSESSMENT

A. CARDIOVASCULAR ANGINA 0 ARRHYTHMIA 0 MURMUR 0 EDEMA 0 PALPITATIONS 0

CHEST PAIN 0 MI 0 CVA 0 ANEURYSM 0 HYPERTENSION 0

PACEMAKER 0 TYPE – NO C/O ✓

PULSE STRONG ✓ WEAK ___ REGULAR ✓ IRREGULAR ___

RIGHT DORSALIS PEDAL PULSE STRONG ✓ WEAK ___ ABSENT ___

LEFT DORSALIS PEDAL PULSE STRONG ✓ WEAK ___ ABSENT ___

Figure **2–2.** *(Continued)*

B. RESPIRATORY: COUGH _O_ PRODUCTIVE _O_ PAIN _O_ DESCRIBE _O_

FREQUENT COLDS _O_ HOARSENESS _O_ ASTHMA _O_ TB _O_ SOB: ON EXERTION _O_ AT REST _O_

NO C/O _✓_

COMMENTS _—_

C. RENAL: KIDNEY STONES _O_ INFECTIONS _✓_ RETENTION _O_ BURNING _✓_ POLYURIA _✓_ DYSURIA _✓_

NO C/O _✓_

URINARY DEVICES? _O_ TYPE ____

INCONTINENCE _O_ DAYTIME ____ NOCTURNAL ____ STRESS ____

DO YOU GET UP DURING NIGHT TO URINATE? YES _✓_ NO ____

COMMENTS _Nocturia 1-2 × per night, States he has urinary followup c̄ prostate exam q 1 yr._

D. GASTROINTESTINAL (NUTRITION METABOLIC)

1. HISTORY OF DIABETES? YES ____ NO _✓_ DO YOU TEST FOR SUGAR? YES ____ NO ____ URINE ____ BLOOD ____

DIET CONTROLLED ____ INSULIN DEPENDENT ____ ORAL HYPOGLYCEMICS ____

NUMBER OF YEARS ____ PREVIOUS DIABETES EDUCATION YES ____ NO ____

2. NUMBER OF MEALS DAY _3_ SNACKS _1-2_ SPECIAL DIET _O_

3. PATIENT'S ABILITY TO EAT INDEPENDENT _✓_ WITH ASSISTANCE ____ SPECIFY ____

DIFFICULTY SWALLOWING ____

4. WEIGHT CHANGE IN THE LAST SIX MONTHS NONE _✓_ LOST ____ LBS GAINED____ LBS

5. DO YOU EXPERIENCE NAUSEA VOMITING? YES ____ NO _✓_ RELATED TO ____

6. DO YOU EXPERIENCE CRAMPING _NO_ HEARTBURN _occ_ RECTAL PAIN _NO_ GAS _NO_ LAST BM _Yesterday_

7. BOWEL: USUAL TIME _7_ (A.M.)____ P.M. FREQUENCY: DAILY _✓_ EVERY OTHER DAY ____ OTHER ____

INCONTINENCE _O_ DEVICES USED _O_

COLOR: BROWN _✓_ CLAY-COLORED ____ BLACK ____ BLOOD ____

CONSTIPATION: NONE _✓_ OCCASIONALLY ____ FREQUENTLY ____

DIARRHEA: NONE ____ OCCASIONALLY _✓_ FREQUENTLY ____ OSTOMY ____

LAXATIVES/ENEMAS USED HOW OFTEN? (SPECIFY) _O_

8. ABDOMEN SOFT _✓_ NON TENDER ____ NON DISTENDED ____ FIRM ____ TENDER ____ DISTENDED ____

BOWEL SOUNDS PRESENT _✓_ ABSENT ____

COMMENTS _Occasional heartburn – relieved by antacid_

E. SKIN CONDITION

COLOR WNL _✓_ PALE ____ CYANOTIC ____ JAUNDICE ____ OTHER ____

TEMP WARM _✓_ COOL ____ TURGOR WNL _✓_ POOR ____

EDEMA NO _✓_ YES ____ DESCRIPTION LOCATION ____

LESIONS NO _✓_ YES ____ DESCRIPTION LOCATION ____

DECUBITUS NO _✓_ YES ____ LOCATIONS ____ (SEE TISSUE TRAUMA FORM)

BRUISES NO _✓_ YES ____ DESCRIPTION LOCATION ____

RASHES NO _✓_ YES ____ DESCRIPTION LOCATION ____

REDNESS NO _✓_ YES ____ DESCRIPTION LOCATION ____

COMMENTS _Healthy skin_

Figure **2–2.** *(Continued)*

F. MUSCULO-SKELETAL CRAMPING 0 ARTHRITIS 0 STIFFNESS 0 SWELLING 0 NO C/O See below

MOTOR FUNCTION RIGHT ARM WNL ✓ AMPUTATED __ SPASTIC __ FLACCID __ WEAKNESS __ PARALYSIS __ OTHER __

LEFT ARM WNL ✓ AMPUTATED __ SPASTIC __ FLACCID __ WEAKNESS __ PARALYSIS __ OTHER __

RIGHT LEG WNL ✓ AMPUTATED __ SPASTIC __ FLACCID __ WEAKNESS __ PARALYSIS __ OTHER __

LEFT LEG WNL ✓ AMPUTATED __ SPASTIC __ FLACCID __ WEAKNESS __ PARALYSIS __ OTHER __

COMMENTS Occasional backache p̄ driving long distances.

VII. SLEEP-REST ACTIVITY

A. USUAL SLEEP PATTERN BEDTIME 11³⁰p HOURS SLEPT 6–8 NAPS NO ✓ YES __

B. DIFFICULTY FALLING ASLEEP NO ✓ YES __ SPECIFY Occasional insomnia

C. SLEEP AIDS USED NO ✓ YES __ SPECIFY __

D. DOES PATIENT HAVE DIFFICULTY/PROBLEMS IN:

BATHING NO ✓ YES __ SPECIFY __

DRESSING NO ✓ YES __ SPECIFY __

AMBULATING NO ✓ YES __ BALANCE/GAIT: STEADY __ UNSTEADY __ TIRES EASILY __ WEAKNESS __

COMMENTS Self-sufficient

VIII. SEXUAL HEALTH

A. LMP __ LAST PAP SMEAR __

B. DO YOU EXAMINE YOUR BREASTS/(TESTICLES)? YES __ NO ✓ HOW OFTEN? __

C. IF NO, DO YOU KNOW HOW? YES __ NO ✓ WOULD YOU BE INTERESTED IN LEARNING? YES ✓ NO __

PAMPHLET GIVEN? YES ✓ NO __ COMMENTS Wants to review pamphlet c̄ physician.

IX. ASSESSMENT SUMMARY: Generally healthy except UTI. Very thirsty – probably dry. Says he's been too sick to drink fluids – just slept a lot.

X. NURSING DIAGNOSES: Fluid Volume Deficit R/T ↑ fluid needs 2° to UTI and fever + poor intake

DISCHARGE PLANNING SHEET INITIATED? YES ✓ NO __

INJURY RISK SHEET INITIATED? YES __ NO ✓

TEACHING PLAN INITIATED? YES __ NO ✓

XI. THE FOLLOWING SECTIONS WERE DEFERRED ON ADMISSION (IDENTIFY BY SECTION NUMBER): None

REASON

DATE TIME	COMPLETED BY	PRIMARY NURSE	DATE TIME	REVIEWED BY PRIMARY NURSE
3/3/98	L Ballard RN	YES ✓ NO __		RN

Figure 2–2. *(Continued)*

Community Nursing Service & Hospice

NURSING EVALUATION

EXPECTED OUTCOME	RANKING KEY
1. Normal	
2. Abnormal but stable	
3. Abnormal but improved	
4. Abnormal	

CLIENT'S NAME ____________

FID# ____________

FUNDING SOURCE: (CHECK ONE)
☐ MEDICARE ☐ PRIVATE INS.
☐ MEDICAID ☐ SELF-PAY
☐ OTHER ____________
BRANCH ____________

____ Certification ____ Recertification **PERIOD: FROM** ____________ **TO** ____________

Reason for referral (admission only): ____________

☐ Y ☐ N HOLD 485 for other disciplines? WHO? ☐ P.T. ☐ O.T. ☐ S.T. ☐ OTHER ____________

☐ Y ☐ N DELETE 485 information from other disciplines? WHO? ☐ P.T. ☐ O.T. ☐ S.T. ☐ OTHER ____________

RN SIGNATURE ____________ DATE ____________ Casemanager? ☐ YES ☐ NO

Casemanager (if known): ____________

EXPECTED OUTCOME	1	2	3	4

R L L R

INTEGUMENT: ☐ History: ____________
☐ Jaundice
☐ Petechiae
☐ Rashes
☐ Lesions
☐ Contusions Why ____________
☐ Wound/pressure sore
size L____ (see
W____ drawing)
D____
☐ Suture line ____________
☐ Drainage ____________
☐ Other ____________
☐ No problems

INTERVENTION: ☐ No ☐ Yes
Who ____________ Why ____________

EXPECTED OUTCOME	1	2	3	4

PAIN: ☐ History: ____________
Location ____________
Intensity (scale 1-10) ____________
Quality ____________
Frequency ____________
Relief ____________
☐ No problems

INTERVENTION: ☐ No ☐ Yes
Who ____________
Why ____________
Methods ____________

EXPECTED OUTCOME	1	2	3	4

NEUROMUSCULAR: ☐ History: ____________
☐ Weakness
☐ Impaired balance
☐ Impaired use of hands
☐ Paresthesias
☐ Hernia
☐ No problems
☐ Impaired gait/ROM
☐ Seizures ____________
☐ Tremors ____________
☐ Paralysis ____________
☐ Developmental delay
☐ Normal reflexes

INTERVENTION: ☐ No ☐ Yes Who ____________
Why ____________

EXPECTED OUTCOME	1	2	3	4

CNS132 (6/92)

TRANSCRIPTION COPY
TRAVELING COPY

Figure 2–3. (Courtesy of Community Nursing Service, Salt Lake City, Utah.

CLIENT'S NAME ____________

FID# ____________

2

FUNCTIONAL LIMITATIONS:

☐ 1 Amputation
☐ 2 Bowel/Bladder
☐ 3 Contracture
☐ 4 Hearing
☐ 5 Paralysis
☐ Infant
☐ B Other ____________
☐ 6 Endurance
☐ 7 Ambulation
☐ 8 Speech
☐ 9 Legally blind
☐ A Dyspnea with minimal exertion

ADL LIMITATIONS AND PRIOR FUNCTIONAL STATUS: ____________

ACTIVITIES PERMITTED:

☐ 1 Bedrest complete
☐ 2 Bedrest BRP
☐ 3 Up as tolerated
☐ 4 Transfer bed/chair
☐ 5 Exercise prescribed
☐ 6 Partial weight bear
☐ 7 Independent at home
☐ 8 Crutches ☐ 9 Cane
☐ A Wheelchair
☐ B Walker
☐ C No restrictions
☐ D Other ____________
☐ Infant

MENTAL STATUS:

☐ 1 Oriented
☐ 2 Comatose
☐ 3 Forgetful
☐ 4 Depressed
☐ 5 Disoriented
☐ 6 Lethargic
☐ 7 Agitated
☐ 8 Other ____________

PROGNOSIS: ☐ 1 Poor ☐ 2 Guarded ☐ 3 Fair ☐ 4 Good ☐ 5 Excellent

REHAB POTENTIAL: ☐ Full recovery/independent of CNS Care ☐ Return to preacute level
☐ Will require ongoing CNS care ☐ Endstage illness, support until death
Other ____________

ALLERGIES: ____________

SELF-CARE:	FEEDING	MEAL PREP	BATH/ PERS. CARE	DRESSING/ GROOMING	TRANS-FERS	AMBUL-LATION	TOILET-ING	HOUSE-KEEPING	LAUNDRY SHOPPING	MANG. FIN.
IND.	☐	☐	☐	☐	☐	☐	☐	☐	☐	☐
MECH. ASST.	☐	☐	☐	☐	☐	☐	☐	☐	☐	☐
MOD. ASST.	☐	☐	☐	☐	☐	☐	☐	☐	☐	☐
DEP.	☐	☐	☐	☐	☐	☐	☐	☐	☐	☐

INTERVENTION: ☐ No ☐ Yes Who ____________ Why ____________

EXPECTED OUTCOME	1	2	3	4

☐ CLIENT/S.O. IS INVOLVED IN CAREPLANNING. Who ____________

CAREGIVER CAPABILITY ☐ Suff. ☐ Ltd. ☐ Inconsistent ☐ None

CARDIOVASCULAR: ____________

☐ History ____________
☐ Edema - Degree ______ Where ______ When ______
Cap. Refill ______ secs
Pedal Pulses R ______ L ______
☐ Chest Pain ___ c̄ ___ s̄ activity
Degree ______ Frequency ______
Duration ______ Relief ______
Other ____________
Cyanosis - Where ____________
☐ Murmurs
☐ Orthopnea
☐ Palpitations
☐ Bleeding Problems ____________
☐ S/S Orthostatic Hypotension ____________
☐ Cardiopulmonary monitor ____________
☐ Juglar Venous Distention
☐ No problem

INTERVENTION: ☐ No ☐ Yes Who ____________
Why ____________

EXPECTED OUTCOME	1	2	3	4

RESPIRATORY: ____________

☐ History ____________
Lung Sounds ____________
☐ SOB ☐ c̄ ☐ s̄ exertion
☐ Cough ______ Retractions
☐ Sputum Color ____________
Amt ____________
☐ Smoker Amt ______ Yrs ______
☐ 02 ____ l/min per
☐ Other equipment ____________
☐ Other ____________
☐ No problems

INTERVENTION: ☐ No ☐ Yes
Who ____________
Why ____________

EXPECTED OUTCOME	1	2	3	4

CNS132 (6/92)

TRANSCRIPTION COPY
TRAVELING COPY

Figure **2–3.** *(Continued)*

CLIENT'S NAME ______
FID# ______

3

GI

☐ History ______
Last BM ______
Bowel Habits ______
☐ Constipation
☐ Diarrhea
☐ Incontinence
☐ N/V
☐ Rectal bleeding
☐ Indigestion
☐ Appetite
☐ Hydration
☐ Ascites ______
☐ Liver involvement
☐ Breast feeding
☐ Bottle feeding
amount ______
☐ Other ______
☐ No problems
INTERVENTION: ☐ No ☐ Yes
Who ______
Why ______

EXPECTED OUTCOME	1	2	3	4

GU

☐ History ______
Uninary Habits ______
☐ Incontinent ___ diapers ___ pads
☐ Indwelling Cath size ___ fr
freq. of change ______
☐ Condom cath ___ Circumcision
☐ Frequency ___ Urgency ___ Hesitancy
☐ Nocturia ___ Dysuria
☐ Pyuria ___ Hematuria
☐ Other ______
☐ No problems

INTERVENTION: ☐ No ☐ Yes
Who ______
Why ______

EXPECTED OUTCOME	1	2	3	4

ENDOCRINE

☐ History ______
☐ Hyperthyroid
☐ Hypothyroid
☐ Pancreas
☐ IDDM ☐ NIDDM
☐ PBS ______
☐ Prostate
☐ Uterus
☐ Breast Lumps
☐ Discharge
☐ Performs SBE
☐ Other ______
☐ No problems
INTERVENTION: ☐ No ☐ Yes
Who ______
Why ______

EXPECTED OUTCOME	1	2	3	4

NUTRITIONAL REQUIREMENTS:
______
______

EYES/EARS/NOSE/THROAT ☐ History ______

☐ Vision Impairment
☐ Glasses ☐ Contacts
☐ Can ☐ Cannot see print
☐ Can ☐ Cannot see television
☐ Can ☐ Cannot see shadows
☐ Legally blind
☐ Inflammation ☐ Discharge
☐ Cataracts ☐ Glaucoma
☐ No problems

☐ Hearing impairment
☐ Hearing aides ☐ L ☐ R
☐ Vertigo
☐ Tinnitus
☐ Other ______
☐ No problems

☐ Sinus problems
☐ Nosebleeds
frequency ______
☐ Discharge
☐ Patent ☐ R ☐ L
☐ Other ______
☐ No problem

☐ Hoarseness ☐ Dysphagia ☐ Difficulty chewing
☐ Mouth sores/irritation/bleeding ☐ Dentures ☐ upper ☐ lower ☐ partial ______
Mouth breather ☐ Poor suck response ☐ No problem

INTERVENTION: ☐ No ☐ Yes Who ______ Why ______

EXPECTED OUTCOME	1	2	3	4

DME AND SUPPLIES: ______
______
______

REASON HOMEBOUND: ______
______

MEDICAL/NON-MEDICAL REASONS CLIENT REGULARLY LEAVES HOME AND HOW OFTEN:
______

CNS132 (6/92)

TRANSCRIPTION COPY
TRAVELING COPY

Figure **2–3.** *(Continued)*

CLIENT'S NAME ____________________

FID# ____________________

4

PSYCHOSOCIAL:
CIRCLE ONE
(Y = Yes N = No)

	CLIENT		SO/WHO ________	
Cooperative	Y	N	Y	N
Willing/capable of learning	Y	N	Y	N
Communication impairment	Y	N	Y	N
Speech impairment	Y	N	Y	N
Impaired comprehension	Y	N	Y	N
Language barrier	Y	N	Y	N
Depressed	Y	N	Y	N
Anxiety	Y	N	Y	N
Grief	Y	N	Y	N
Combative	Y	N	Y	N
Hostile	Y	N	Y	N
Agitated	Y	N	Y	N
Confused	Y	N	Y	N
Interpersonal conflict	Y	N	Y	N
Illiterate	Y	N	Y	N

CLIENT'S STATEMENT OF EXPECTATIONS/OUTCOME OF HOME CARE:
____
____
____

INTERVENTION: ☐ No ☐ Yes
Who ____________________
Why ____________________

EXPECTED OUTCOME	1	2	3	4

LIVING ARRANGEMENTS:
☐ A. Lives alone ☐ home ☐ apt.
☐ B. Lives with willing persons
☐ family ☐ friends
☐ C. Lives with unwilling persons
☐ D. Other

UNUSUAL HOME/SOCIAL ENVIRONMENT:
____
____
____

ASSISTANCE FROM RELATIVES/FRIENDS:
(Support systems) ____________________
____
____
____

IS CLIENT RECIEVING CARE PAID FOR BY OTHER THAN MEDICARE? ☐ YES ☐ NO Who ________
No. of people in household ______ Teach family/S.O. ☐ YES ☐ NO
Approx. length of care ____________________
ANY SUPPLEMENTARY TREATMENT PLANS FROM OTHER THAN REFERRING PHYSICIAN? ☐ YES ☐ NO
(Refer to orders)

Desires Home care ☐ Yes ☐ No

SAFETY: (✓ = Assessed += problem) CIRCLE ONE

+ ✓ Home safe	+ ✓ Cluttered	+ ✓ Food adequate
+ ✓ Telephone	+ ✓ Pests	+ ✓ Heat adequate
+ ✓ Running Water	+ ✓ Pets	+ ✓ Bedding adequate
+ ✓ Electricity	+ ✓ Stairs # ______	+ ✓ Lighting
+ ✓ Refrigerator	where ______	+ ✓ Able to call for help
+ ✓ Handrails	+ ✓ Elevator	+ ✓ Safe neighborhood

COMMUNITY RESOURCES
☐ County mental health
☐ MOW
☐ Transportation
☐ Alternatives
☐ WIC
☐ Sr. companion
☐ Other ________

INTERVENTION: ☐ No ☐ Yes Who ____________________ Why ____________________

CLIENT IS SAFE AT HOME WITH SERVICES CNS CAN PROVIDE: ☐ Yes ☐ No

CNS132 (6/92)

TRANSCRIPTION COPY
TRAVELING COPY

Figure **2–3.** *(Continued)*

DISPLAY 2–1 Federal Government Requirements Influencing Data Base Assessment*

Omnibus Budget Reconciliation Act of 1987: To improve standards of long-term care, the government passed legislation that mandates that certain information be recorded on nursing assessments.

All long-term care facilities receiving Medicare and Medicaid reimbursement must:

- Design a comprehensive and accurate assessment system that is standardized and reproducible. These assessments are the basis for identifying problems and strengths and for developing an individualized care plan that aims to attain the highest physical, mental, and psychosocial functioning.
- Collect a minimum set of data (known as minimum data set, or MDS) in a standardized way (see Fig. 2–4 on p. 44, which shows the first page of the MDS).

---

*From: Alfaro-LeFevre workshop handouts © 1995.

Focus Assessment

Focus assessments are often performed to monitor specific problems. Below are some questions you should ask when collecting data to focus on the status of a specific problem.

- What evidence do I have that indicates that this problem exists right now? Compared with the baseline data (data gathered before treatment began), does the evidence indicate that the problem is better, worse, or the same?
- What factors are contributing to the problem, and what's been done about these factors?
- How does the person feel about managing or preventing the problem? Is he or she able to explain how to manage or prevent the problem?

Display 2–2 shows how to apply these questions to assessing *Constipation.*

DISPLAY 2–2 Focus Assessment for Constipation

1. **Do I have evidence that indicates** *Constipation* (eg, no recent bowel movement; hard, dry stool; abdominal cramping; difficulty passing stool)? Compared to the baseline data, does this evidence indicate that the constipation is better, worse, or the same?
2. **What factors are contributing to the** *Constipation* (eg, poor diet, lack of fluid intake, medication side effects, immobility)? How can we ensure a good diet with enough roughage and fluid intake? Is there anything we can do about the immobility? What can we do about medication side effects? Would laxatives help? How can we be sure we stay on top of this problem?
3. **How does the person feel about preventing and managing** *Constipation?* Is he able to relate how to do this? Do I need to do some teaching?

The Nursing Interview and Physical Assessment

Interviews and physical assessments complement and clarify one another. For example, note the following example showing how information gained from a physical examination complements and clarifies information gathered from an interview.

EXAMPLE

> You interview someone who tells you, "I feel like my breathing isn't quite right, but I can't explain exactly what I mean." You then take a stethoscope and listen to her lungs. What you hear (whether the lung sounds are normal or abnormal) gives you additional information that helps you determine breathing status because it complements and clarifies what you've been told.

Ethical, Cultural, and Spiritual Considerations

The success of your interviewing and examination techniques is influenced by your awareness of ethical, cultural, and spiritual concerns. As a nurse, you must:

1. Provide services with respect for human dignity and the uniqueness of the client, unrestricted by considerations of social or economic status, personal attributes, or the nature of health problems (ANA, 1985).

2. Safeguard the client's right to privacy by judiciously protecting information of a confidential nature (ANA, 1985).

3. Be honest. Tell the person the truth about how you'll use the data (eg, "I have to write a paper examining someone's eating patterns. Would you be willing to tell me about your eating habits?").

4. Respect individual cultural and religious beliefs, and be aware of physical tendencies related to culture. This includes being aware of:

   Biological variations. For example, differences among racial and ethnic groups (eg, skin color and texture, and susceptibility to diseases like hypertension or sickle cell anemia).

   Comfortable communication patterns. For example, be sensitive to such things as how language and gestures are used, whether eye contact or touching is acceptable, and whether the person is threatened by being in close proximity to another.

   Family organization and practices. We have diverse family units and practices we must understand to gain insight into factors that influence health status.

   Beliefs about whether people are able to control nature and influence their ability to be healthy (eg, whether blood transfusions are allowed, whether rituals are required).

   The person's concept of "God" and beliefs about the relationship between spiritual beliefs and health status (eg, "God gives you what you deserve").

The Nursing Interview

Your ability to establish rapport, ask questions, listen, and observe is the key to a positive nurse–patient relationship and essential to getting the facts. People who seek health care, whether they're well or acutely ill, are in an extremely vulnerable position; they need to know that they're in good hands and that their main concerns will be addressed. This is where you come in. Consider the guidelines below that can help you perform an interview that establishes trust, instills confidence, creates a positive attitude, and reduces anxiety.

Guidelines: Promoting a Caring Interview

How to Establish Rapport

- Before you go into the interview
    - **Get organized:** When you know what you're going to do, you're more confident and able to focus on the person.
    - **Don't rely on memory:** Have a written or printed plan to guide the questions you'll be asking. Some nurses use the nursing data base as a guide (see Figure 2–4).
    - **Plan enough time:** The admission interview usually takes ½ to 1 hour.
    - **Ensure privacy:** Make sure you have a quiet, private setting, free from interruptions or distractions.
    - **Get focused:** Take a minute to clear your mind of other concerns (other duties, worries about yourself). Say to yourself, "getting to know this person is the most important thing I have to do right now."
    - **Visualize yourself as being confident, warm, and helpful:** Seeing yourself in this light helps you to *be* confident, warm, and helpful; your genuine interest comes through.
- When you begin the interview
    - **Give the person your name and position** (if the person can read, give it in writing). This sends the message that you accept responsibility and are willing to be accountable for your actions.
    - **Verify the person's name and ask what he or she would like to be called** (eg, "I have your name listed here as Michael Riley. Is that correct? What would you like us to call you?"). Verifying the name sends the message that you want to make sure things are correct. Using the preferred name helps the person feel more relaxed and sends the message that you recognize that this person is an individual who has likes and dislikes.
    - **Briefly explain your purpose** (eg, "I'm here to do the admission interview to help us plan your nursing care").
- During the interview
    - **Give the person your full attention:** Avoid the impulse to become engrossed in your notes or reading the assessment tool.
    - **Don't hurry:** Rushing sends the message that you're not interested in what the person has to say.

MDS Form

MINIMUM DATA SET FOR NURSING HOME RESIDENT ASSESSMENT AND CARE SCREENING (MDS)

(Status in last 7 days, unless other time frame indicated)

SECTION A. IDENTIFICATION AND BACKGROUND INFORMATION

1.	ASSESSMENT DATE	__ __ – __ __ – __ __ __ __ Month Day Year
2.	RESIDENT NAME	(First) (Middle Initial) (Last)
3.	SOCIAL SECURITY NO.	__ __ __ – __ __ – __ __ __ __
4.	MEDICAID NO. (If applicable)	
5.	MEDICAL RECORD NO.	
6.	REASON FOR ASSESS-MENT	1. Initial admission assess. 2. Hosp/Medicare reassess. 3. Readmission assessment 4. Annual assessment 5. Significant change in status 6. Other (e.g., UR)
7.	CURRENT PAYMENT SOURCE(S) FOR N.H. STAY	*(Billing Office to indicate; check all that apply)* Medicaid a. Medicare b. CHAMPUS c. VA d. Self pay/Private insurance e. Other f.
8.	RESPONSI-BILITY/ LEGAL GUARDIAN	*(Check all that apply)* Legal guardian a. Other legal oversight b. Durable power attrny./health care proxy c. Family member responsible d. Resident responsible e. *NONE OF ABOVE* f.
9.	ADVANCED DIRECTIVES	*(For those items with supporting documentation in the medical record, check all that apply)* Living will a. Do not resuscitate b. Do not hospitalize c. Organ donation d. Autopsy request e. Feeding restrictions f. Medication restrictions g. Other treatment restrictions h. *NONE OF ABOVE* i.
10.	DISCHARGE PLANNED WITHIN 3 MOS.	*(Does not include discharge due to death)* 0. No 1. Yes 2. Unknown/uncertain
11.	PARTICIPATE IN ASSESS-MENT	a. Resident 0. No 1. Yes; b. Family 0. No 1. Yes 2. No family
12.	SIGNATURES	Signature of RN Assessment Coordinator; Signatures of Others Who Completed Part of the Assessment

SECTION B. COGNITIVE PATTERNS

1.	COMATOSE	*(Persistent vegetative state/no discernible consciousness)* 0. No 1. Yes *(Skip to SECTION E)*
2.	MEMORY	*(Recall of what was learned or known)* a. Short-term memory OK—seems/appears to recall after 5 minutes 0. Memory OK 1. Memory problem; b. Long-term memory OK—seems/appears to recall long past 0. Memory OK 1. Memory problem
3.	MEMORY/ RECALL ABILITY	*(Check all that resident normally able to recall during last 7 days)* Current season a. Location of own room b. Staff names/faces c. That he/she is in a nursing home d. *NONE OF ABOVE* are recalled e.
4.	COGNITIVE SKILLS FOR DAILY DECISION-MAKING	*(Made decisions regarding tasks of daily life)* 0. Independent—decisions consistent/reasonable 1. Modified Independence—some difficulty in new situations only 2. Moderately Impaired—decisions poor; cues/supervision required 3. Severely Impaired—never/rarely made decisions
5.	INDICATORS OF DELIRIUM —PERIODIC DISORDERED THINKING/ AWARENESS	*(Check if condition over last 7 days appears different from usual functioning)* Less alert, easily distracted a. Changing awareness of environment b. Episodes of incoherent speech c. Periods of motor restlessness or lethargy d. Cognitive ability varies over course of day e. *NONE OF ABOVE* f.
6.	CHANGE IN COGNITIVE STATUS	Change in resident's cognitive status, skills, or abilities in last 90 days 0. No change 1. Improved 2. Deteriorated

SECTION C. COMMUNICATION/HEARING PATTERNS

1.	HEARING	*(With hearing appliance, if used)* 0. Hears adequately—normal talk, TV, phone 1. Minimal difficulty when not in quiet setting 2. Hears in special situations only—speaker has to adjust tonal quality and speak distinctly 3. Highly impaired/absence of useful hearing
2.	COMMUNI-CATION DEVICES/ TECHNIQUES	*(Check all that apply during last 7 days)* Hearing aid, present and used a. Hearing aid, present and not used b. Other receptive comm. techniques used (e.g., lip read) c. *NONE OF ABOVE* d.
3.	MODES OF EXPRESSION	*(Check all used by resident to make needs known)* Speech a. Writing messages to express or clarify needs b. Signs/gestures/sounds c. Communication board d. Other e. *NONE OF ABOVE* f.
4.	MAKING SELF UNDER-STOOD	*(Express information content—however able)* 0. Understood 1. Usually Understood—difficulty finding words or finishing thoughts 2. Sometimes Understood—ability is limited to making concrete requests 3. Rarely/Never Understood
5.	ABILITY TO UNDER-STAND OTHERS	*(Understanding verbal information content—however able)* 0. Understands 1. Usually Understands—may miss some part/intent of message 2. Sometimes Understands—responds adequately to simple, direct communication 3. Rarely/Never Understands
6.	CHANGE IN COMMUNI-CATION/ HEARING	Resident's ability to express, understand or hear information has changed over last 90 days 0. No change 1. Improved 2. Deteriorated

SECTION D. VISION PATTERNS

1.	VISION	*(Ability to see in adequate light and with glasses if used)* 0. Adequate—sees fine detail, including regular print in newspapers/books 1. Impaired—sees large print, but not regular print in newspapers/books 2. Highly Impaired—limited vision; not able to see newspaper headlines; appears to follow objects with eyes 3. Severely Impaired—no vision or appears to see only light, colors, or shapes
2.	VISUAL LIMITATIONS/ DIFFICULTIES	Side vision problems—decreased peripheral vision (e.g., leaves food on one side of tray, difficulty traveling, bumps into people and objects, misjudges placement of chair when seating self) a. Experiences any of following: sees halos or rings around lights; sees flashes of light; sees "curtains" over eyes b. *NONE OF ABOVE* c.
3.	VISUAL APPLIANCES	Glasses; contact lenses; lens implant; magnifying glass 0. No 1. Yes

▒ = Code the appropriate response ☐ = Check all the responses that apply

Appendix B: Page B-2 December, 1990

Figure 2–4. The first page of the Minimum Data Set (developed by HCFA).

How to Listen

- **Be an empathetic listener** (see page 24)
- **Use short supplementary phrases** that let the person know you understand and encourage the person to continue. Some examples are, "I see," "mm-hm," "oh, no," "and . . . ," and "then what?" A nod of the head also lets the person know you're listening.
- **Listen for feelings** as well as words. For example, the person who sighs, looks away, and says, "I think I'll be okay with this," might be telling you, "I doubt this is going to work."
- **Let the person know when you see body language that sends a message that conflicts with what is being said** (eg, "You say that you aren't having pain, but you look uncomfortable to me").
- **Allow the person to finish sentences.** Be calm and don't rush him.
- **Be patient if the person has a memory block.** This information may be remembered later when you ask related questions.
- **Avoid the impulse to interrupt.** If the interview is getting off track, allow the person to finish his sentence, then say, "We seem to be getting off track; can we get back to . . . ?"
- **Allow for pauses in conversation**. Silence gives both you and the person time to gather thoughts.

How to Ask Questions

- **Ask about the person's main problem first** (eg, "What is the main reason you're here today?").
- **Focus your questions to gain specific information about signs and symptoms.** For example: "Show me where the problem is. Can you describe how this feels more specifically? When did this start? When does this seem to happen? Is there anything that makes it better? What makes it worse?"
- **Don't use leading questions** that are likely to lead the person to a specific response (eg, "You don't drink alcohol, do you?" leads the person to a "no" answer).
- **Do use exploratory statements** (statements that begin with words like *tell, describe, explain,* and *elaborate*) to direct the person to tell you more about a specific condition (eg, "Tell me more about your sleeping patterns").*
- **Use communication techniques that enhance your ability to think critically and get the facts:**
  - Use phrases that help you see the other person's perspective (eg, "From your point of view, what are the biggest problems?" or "What are the problems as you see them?").
  - Restate the person's own words. This clarifies meaning and encourages the person to expand on what's been said (eg, "When you say . . . , what are you saying?" or "When you say . . . , does this mean . . . ?").

---

* Some authors call these types of statements *leading statements*. I use *exploratory statements* to avoid confusion with leading questions, which shouldn't be used.

  - Ask open-ended questions (questions requiring more than a one-word answer, such as "How are you feeling?" rather than "Are you feeling well?").
- **Avoid closed-ended questions** (those requiring a one-word answer) unless the person is too ill to elaborate or you're trying to clarify a response by getting a yes or no answer. The following are some examples of appropriate use of closed-ended questions: Asking someone who is short of breath, "Are you having pain?" Asking, "You've told me you've had pain for 2 weeks, but not all the time. Are you saying it comes and goes?" Asking, "Is there a history of hypertension in your family?"

Display 2–3 gives more examples of open-ended and closed-ended questions. Table 2–1 summarizes the advantages and disadvantages of using each of these types of questions.

How to Observe

- **Use your senses.** Do you see, hear, or smell anything abnormal?
- **Notice general appearance.** Does the person appear well groomed, healthy, well nourished?
- **Observe body language.** Does the person appear comfortable? Nervous? Withdrawn? Apprehensive? What behaviors do you see?
- **Notice interaction patterns**. Be aware of the person's responses to your interviewing style (eg, sometimes cultural and personal differences create communication barriers).

How to Terminate the Interview

- **Ask the person to summarize her most important concerns**, then summarize the most important concerns as you see them. For example, say, "OK, we've talked about a lot of things. To make sure I have it right, tell me the most important things I can help you with."
- **Offer yourself as a resource.** Explain that you expect that new needs may arise and that you'd like to be kept informed so you can make changes as necessary.

DISPLAY 2–3 Examples of Open-Ended and Closed-Ended Questions

✓ **Closed-Ended:** "Are you happy about this?"
✓ **Open-Ended:** "How does this make you feel?"
✓ **Closed-Ended:** "Do you get along with your husband?"
✓ **Open-Ended:** "What is your relationship with your husband like?"
✓ **Closed-Ended:** "Does this make you sick to your stomach?"
✓ **Open-Ended:** "Describe the feeling that you are experiencing."

TABLE 2–1 Advantages and Disadvantages of Open-Ended and Closed-Ended Questions

Advantages	Disadvantages
Open-Ended Question	
Brings forth more information than a question that requires only a one-word response.	May allow the person to sidestep the question.
Gives people a chance to verbalize and involves them in dialogue.	Requires a more wordy response. This may be undesirable in an emergency situation or if the individual is confused, in pain, or having difficulty breathing.
Tends to bring forth a more honest reply.	Allows opportunity to ramble and get off the track.
Usually less threatening and less likely to convey negative judgment.	
Often interpreted to imply sincere interest.	
Closed-Ended Question	
Helps clarify responses to open-ended questions.	May be more threatening.
Saves time in emergency situations.	Limits the amount of information offered.
Can be helpful in focusing the interview on specific data (eg, following a checklist that asks for history of specific illnesses, such as high blood pressure, heart attacks, etc.)	Does not encourage the person to express concerns from his or her point of view.
May be helpful for those who are confused, in pain, or having difficulty breathing.	Does not encourage active dialogue between the nurse and the person.

- **End on a positive note** and encourage the person to become an active participant. For example, "We have a good start here. I want you to be actively involved in making decisions about your care. Don't hesitate to offer suggestions or ask questions at any time."

Display 2–4 on the next page lists common communication errors to avoid.

Physical Assessment

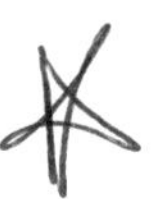

The key to performing a physical assessment is being thorough, systematic, and skilled in technique. Physical assessment skills include the following:

- *Inspection:* Observing carefully by using your fingers, eyes, ears, and sense of smell.
- *Auscultation:* Listening with a stethoscope.
- *Palpation:* Touching and pressing to test for pain and feel inner structures, such as the liver.

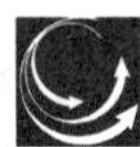

DISPLAY 2-4 Common Communication Errors

- **Using communication techniques you're comfortable with, without observing the response.** For example, some people are uncomfortable with eye contact or use of touch.
- **Using first names without permission.** For some, being called by their first name by someone other than a close friend or family member is a sign of disrespect.
- **Using endearing names.** Most people feel degraded when called "honey, deary, sweetie, pop, grandma" by anyone other than close family.
- **"Talking down."** For example, saying, "So you've had a pain in your tummy?"
- **Using medical terminology with lay people.** Many people don't know common medical terms, such as void, vital signs, BM.

- *Percussion:* Directly or indirectly tapping a body surface to determine reflexes (done with a percussion hammer) or to determine whether an area contains fluid (done by tapping fingers over surface).

The best way to become thorough and systematic in physical assessment is to choose a good way to organize your approach and use it consistently so it becomes automatic.

How you organize your assessment is influenced by two things:

1. **The person's condition:** If the person is ill, begin by examining the area where the problems are before going on to other parts of the body. For example, if there is abdominal pain, you examine the abdomen first; if you find someone unconscious, you assess according to the ABCs (airway, breathing, circulation) of cardiopulmonary resuscitation (CPR).
2. **Your own preference:** For example, you may choose a head-to-toe approach, beginning by assessing the head and neck, continuing down the body to the thorax, abdomen, legs, and feet, in that order. Or you may choose a systems approach, starting with the respiratory system (nose, mouth, throat, lungs) and continuing with cardiac, circulatory, neurologic, gastrointestinal, genitourinary, musculoskeletal, and skin status.

The following guidelines can help you develop habits that promote a thorough and systematic physical assessment.

Guidelines: Performing a Physical Assessment

- **Promote communication between yourself and the person you're examining.** Provide for privacy, establish rapport, and use good interviewing techniques (rather than working in silence).
- **Don't rely on memory.** Jot down notes to be sure of accuracy.
- **Choose a method of organizing your assessment** and use it consistently. For example, use the method listed below, which expands on the ABCs of CPR.

- **Respiratory status:** Airway, breath sounds, rate and depth of breathing, cough, symmetry, presence of pain/discomfort.
- **Cardiac status:** Apical rate, rhythm, heart sounds, presence of pain/discomfort.
- **Circulatory status:** Rate, rhythm, and quality of pulses (radial, brachial, carotid, femoral, dorsalis pedis); presence of pain/discomfort.
- **Neurologic status:** Mental status; orientation; pupillary reaction; vision and appearance of the eyes; gag reflex; ability to hear, taste, feel, and smell; gait; coordination; presence of pain/discomfort.
- **Skin status:** Color, temperature, turgor, edema, lesions, hair distribution, presence of itching/pain/discomfort.
- **Musculoskeletal status:** Muscle tone, strength, range of motion, presence of pain/ discomfort.
- **Gastrointestinal status:** Condition of the lips, tongue, gums, teeth; presence of bowel sounds; presence of abdominal distention or tenderness; impaction; hemorrhoids.
- **Genitourinary status:** Color and amount of urine, presence of distended bladder, discharge (vaginal, urethral), presence of pain/discomfort; (for women) breast examination, condition of the vulva; (for men) testicular examination.

Checking Laboratory and Diagnostic Studies

Checking laboratory and diagnostic studies is essential to performing a comprehensive assessment. These studies are like a "report card" on how the body is functioning. They often provide key evidence that helps you determine health status. For example, you may have perfectly normal assessment data, then note a low potassium level, which needs evaluation and treatment because it creates a risk for cardiac arrhythmias. Or you may have some suspicions about the presence of a health problem, such as dehydration, that may be confirmed by laboratory studies, such as a high hematocrit.

PRACTICE SESSION III

The Nursing Interview and Physical Assessment

To complete this session, read pages 30–49. Example responses can be found on page 231.

Part One: The Interview

1. **Practice making open-ended questions.** Restate each question below so it's an open-ended question.

   a. "Are you feeling better?"

   Tell me how your feeling

b. "Did you like dinner?"

How was your dinner?

c. "Are you happy here?"

How do you feel about beinghere?

d. "Are you having pain?"

Tell me how your feling

2. **Practice clarifying ideas by using reflection (restating what you hear) and making open-ended questions.** For each statement below, write a reflective statement and an open-ended question that would help you to clarify what has been said.

   a. "I've been sick off and on for a month."

   b. "Nothing ever goes right for me."

   c. "I seem to have a pain in my side that comes and goes."

   d. "I've had this funny feeling for a week."

3. **Test your knowledge of communication techniques.** Read each sentence below and identify whether it is an open-ended statement (O), a closed-ended statement (C), a leading question (L), an exploratory statement (E), or a supplementary phrase or statement intended to help the person continue (S).

   a. ___C___ Are you afraid of dying?

   b. ___E___ Tell me when this first started.

   c. ___S___ I see.

d. __L__ You're not still afraid to feed Susan, are you?
e. __O__ How do you think you'll be doing this at home?
f. __C__ Do you have a history of hypertension in your family?
g. __S__ And . . .?
h. __L__ You do want your family to visit, don't you?
i. __O__ How do you feel about being here?
j. __L__ You don't need more practice, do you?
k. __E__ Explain what you mean by "a long time."

4. Rephrase each leading question you identified above to ask an open-ended question.

Part Two: Physical Assessment

1. Because physical assessment and interviewing go hand-in-hand, use the following situations to practice focusing your interview questions upon areas of concern noted during the physical exam.

   a. You examine and find: the patient's hands and fingernails are filthy with ground-in dirt, although the rest of him is clean. You may state or ask:

   b. You examine and find: the patient has a lump on the back of his head. You may state or ask: U feel a lump on the back of your head, How did it happen

   c. You examine and find: the patient's respirations are 40. You may state or ask:

   d. You examine and find: the patient's right eye is red, teary, and inflamed. You may state or ask:

2. Now practice focusing your physical exam on areas of concern voiced by the patient.

   a. Patient states: "I have had a rash that comes and goes." You may reply and examine:

   b. Patient states: "My stomach has been hurting me." You may reply and examine:

   c. Patient states: "I find it burns when I urinate." You may reply and examine:

   d. Patient states: "I feel like I'm heavier than usual, like I'm bloated with fluid." You may reply and examine:

Identifying Subjective and Objective Data

Many nurses find it helpful to separate assessment data into two categories: subjective data (what the person *states*) and objective data (what you *observe*). Separating information into these two categories aids critical thinking because each complements and clarifies the other. For example, your notes might look like this:

Subjective data: States, "I feel like my heart is racing."

Objective data: Pulse 150 beats, regular, and strong.

The objective data above *support* the subjective data: what you observe confirms what the person is stating.

Sometimes what you observe and what the person states are different. For example, your notes might look like this:

Subjective data: States, "I feel fine."

Objective data: Color pale, becomes easily short of breath.

What the person states above *isn't supported* by what you observe. You have to do more investigating to understand the full scope of the problems.

The following can help you remember the difference between these two types of data:

S—S: **S**ubjective data = **S**tated
O—O: **O**bjective data = **O**bserved

Keep in mind that you should chart objective data using as specific (measurable) terms as possible (eg, *a temperature of 100.6°F* is more specific and measurable than *feverish*). Chart subjective data using the person's own words in quotation marks.

Below are some examples of subjective and objective data:

Subjective Data	***Objective Data***
"I feel sick to my stomach."	Blood pressure of 110/70.
"I have a stabbing pain in my side."	Rash on right arm.
"I wish I were home."	Walks with a limp.
"I feel like nobody likes me."	Ate all of his breakfast.
	Urinated 150 mL clear urine.

Identifying Cues and Making Inferences

The subjective and objective data you identify act as *cues*. Cues are data that prompt you to make a judgment, or make an inference, about whether or not a problem may exist. For example, consider the following cues:

Subjective Data: "I just started taking penicillin for a tooth abscess."
Objective Data: Fine rash over trunk.

The above data give you cues that may lead you to infer (suspect) that the person is having an allergic reaction to penicillin. How you interpret or perceive a cue—the conclusion you draw about the cue—is called an *inference*. In this case, you make an inference about the rash: you decide the rash may indicate a penicillin allergy.

Your ability to identify significant cues and make correct inferences is influenced by your observational skills, your nursing knowledge, and your clinical expertise. Your values and beliefs also affect how you interpret certain cues, so make a conscious effort to avoid making value judgments (eg, inferring that a person who bathes only once a week needs to be taught better hygiene, when this practice may be part of his culture).

To clarify your understanding of cues and inferences, study the following examples of cues and corresponding inferences.

Cue: Judy states, "I have trouble moving my bowels."
Inference: Judy may be constipated.

Cue: Jeffrey says he doesn't want to talk and has a sad face.
Inference: Jeffrey may be depressed.
Cue: Mrs. Rayburn's blood pressure is 60/50.
Inference: Mrs. Rayburn is in shock.
Cue: Susan states, "I can't stand this pain any more!"
Inference: Susan is experiencing unbearable pain.

Think About It

Critical thinking requires making judgments based on evidence. When making inferences, or drawing conclusions, the more cues (evidence) you have, the more likely you are to be correct. For example, if you have two cues—the patient just started penicillin and there's a fine rash over the trunk—additional cues, like finding out that the person had a rash before when taking penicillin, can help you confirm what you suspect.

Validating (Verifying) Data

Validating, or verifying that your information is factual and complete, is an essential step in critical thinking. It helps you avoid:

- Making assumptions
- Missing pertinent information
- Misunderstanding situations
- Jumping to conclusions or focusing in the wrong direction
- Making errors in problem identification.

For example, suppose you ask a woman whether she might be pregnant, and she responds, "No." If that's all you ask and you don't verify this by seeking more information (eg, asking *"When was your last period?"* or finding out the results of a pregnancy test), you may operate under the assumption that the woman isn't pregnant, when indeed she is, which can be dangerous. Consider the following guidelines.

Guidelines: Validating (Verifying) Data

- Be aware that data that can be measured accurately can be accepted as factual (eg, height, weight, laboratory study results).*

*There's always the possibility of laboratory error or other factors that may alter the accuracy of the laboratory studies (eg, a fasting blood sugar test that is done even though the person has eaten 1 hour before). Rechecking gross abnormalities should verify whether the studies are valid.

- Keep in mind that data that someone else observes (indirect data) may or may not be true. When the information is critical, verify it by directly observing and interviewing the patient yourself.
- Form the habit of validating data that are questionable by using the following techniques, as appropriate:
  - Double check that your equipment is working correctly.
  - Recheck your own data (eg, take a patient's blood pressure in the opposite arm or 10 minutes later).
  - Look for factors that may alter the accuracy of your data (eg, check whether someone who has an elevated temperature and no other symptoms has just had a hot cup of tea).
  - Ask someone else, preferably an expert, to collect the same data (eg, ask a more experienced nurse to recheck a blood pressure when you're not sure).
  - Always double-check information that's extremely abnormal or inconsistent with patient cues (eg, use two scales to check an infant who appears much heavier or lighter than the scale states; repeat a diagnostic study that is extremely high or low).
  - Compare your subjective and objective data to see if what the person is stating is congruent with what you observe (eg, compare actual pulse rate with perceptions of "racing heart").
  - Clarify statements and verify your inferences (eg, saying, "To me, you seem tired.").
  - Compare your impressions with those of other key members of the health care team.

PRACTICE SESSION IV

Subjective and Objective Data; Cues and Inferences; Validating Data

To complete this session, read pages 52–55. Example responses can be found on page 232.

Part I. Subjective and Objective Data

Case History

Mr. Michaels is 51 years old. He was admitted 2 days ago with chest pain. His physician has ordered the following studies: electrocardiogram, chest x-ray, and complete blood studies including a blood sugar. These studies were just posted on the chart. When you talk with him, he states, "I feel much better today, no more pain. It is a relief to get rid of that discomfort." You think he appears a little tired or weary; he seems to be talking slowly and sighs more often than you think is normal. He denies being weary. His vital signs are:

T: 98.6 P: 74 (regular) R: 22 BP: 140/90

1. List the subjective data noted in the case history above (what were you told directly by Mr. Michaels?).

2. List the objective data noted in the case history above (what information can be readily observed?).

Part II. Cues and Inferences

1. List the cues in the case history above.

2. List the inferences you might make about the cues you've identified.

Part III. Validating Data

1. From the cues and inferences you identified in Part II, indicate in three separate columns those that you feel are *certainly valid, probably valid*, and only *possibly valid*.

2. For the data you list in the *possibly valid* and *probably valid* columns above, identify some methods of clarifying if they are indeed true (eg, what other questions might you ask?).

Try This on Your Own

In a clinical conference or with another student, choose data from a real patient, identify cues, then discuss the inferences you might make from the cues. Discuss how valid the cues and inferences are and how you might clarify or validate the information.

Organizing (Clustering) Data 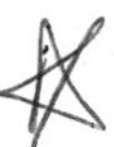

Clustering related data together is a critical-thinking principle that enhances your ability to get a clear picture of health status. Just as putting puzzle pieces with similar colors together helps you see parts of a picture puzzle, clustering health status data into related groups helps you begin to get a picture of various aspects of health status.

If you use a well-designed assessment tool, a lot of the organizing is already complete because the tool guides you to record related cues together (eg, information about nutrition is mostly in one place, information about activity is mostly in one place, and so on). However, because assessment tools don't organize *all* the information, and because ongoing assessment is usually done *without* an assessment tool, this section describes different ways to cluster data for different purposes.

Clustering Data According to a Nursing Model

When identifying nursing diagnoses, it's helpful to cluster data according to a nursing model rather than a medical model. For example, Maslow (1970), Gordon (1994), and Human Response Patterns (NANDA, 1994) offer good ways of clustering data to maintain a nursing focus. (Table 2–2 compares these methods.) These methods are helpful when identifying nursing diagnoses because they're holistic in focus and bring together related data about patterns of human responses and functioning, rather than patterns of organ or system function.

TABLE 2–2 Holistic Models for Clustering Data* (Different methods are used by nurses according to preferences)

Human Needs (Maslow)	Functional Health Patterns (Gordon)	Human Response Patterns (Unitary Person)
Physiologic (survival) needs: Food, fluids, oxygen, elimination, warmth, physical comfort	**Health Perception/Health Management:** Perception of general health status and well-being. Adherence to preventive health practices.	**Exchanging:** Nutritional status, temperature, elimination, oxygenation, circulation, fluid balance, skin and mucous membranes, risks for injury.
Safety and security needs: Things necessary for physical safety (eg, a cane) and psychological security (eg, a child's favorite toy).	**Nutritional-Metabolic:** Patterns of food and fluid intake, fluid and electrolyte balance, general ability to heal.	**Communicating:** Ability to express thoughts verbally; orientation, speech impairments, language barriers.
Love and belonging needs: Family and significant others.	**Elimination:** Patterns of excretory function (bowel, bladder, and skin), and client's perception.	**Relating:** Establishing bonds, social interaction, support systems, role performance (including parenting, occupation, and sexual role).

(Table Continued)

TABLE 2–2 *Continued*

Human Needs (Maslow)	Functional Health* Patterns (Gordon)	Human Response Patterns (Unitary Person)
Self-actualization needs: Need to grow, change, and accomplish goals.	**Activity/Exercise:** Pattern of exercise, activity, leisure, recreation, and ADL; factors that interfere with desired or expected individual pattern. **Cognitive-Perceptual:** Adequacy of sensory modes, such as vision, hearing, taste, touch, smell, pain perception, cognitive functional abilities. **Sleep/Rest:** Patterns of sleep and rest-relaxation periods during 24-hour day, as well as quality and quantity. **Self-Perception/Self-Concept:** Attitudes about self, perception of abilities, body image, identity, general sense of worth and emotional patterns. **Role/Relationship:** Perception of major roles and responsibilities in current life situation. **Sexuality/Reproductive:** Perceived satisfaction or dissatisfaction with sexuality. Reproductive stage and pattern. **Coping/Stress Tolerance:** General coping pattern, stress tolerance, support systems, and perceived ability to control and manage situations. **Value-Belief:** Values, goals, or beliefs that guide choices or decisions.	**Valuing:** Religious and cultural preference and practices, relationship with deity, perception of suffering: acceptance of illness, **Choosing:** Ability to accept help and make decisions, adjustment to health status, desire for independence/dependence, denial of problem, adherence to therapies, **Moving:** Activity tolerance, ability for self-care, sleep patterns, diversional activities, disability history, safety needs, breast feeding. **Perceiving:** Body image, self-esteem, ability to use all five senses, amount of hopefulness, perception of ability to control current situation. **Knowing:** Knowledge about current illness or therapies; previous illnesses; risk factors, expectations of therapy, cognitive abilities; readiness to learn, orientation, memory. **Feeling:** Pain; grieving; risk for violence, anxiety level, emotional integrity.

*From Alfaro-LeFevre workshop handouts © 1995.

Clustering Data According to Body Systems

When identifying data that may indicate a medical problem, the body systems approach (Display 2–5) is helpful because medical problems are caused by abnormalities in system or organ function.

The following diagram shows the relationship between clustering data and identifying health problems.

To be able to recognize medical and nursing problems, be sure to cluster your data both ways—using body systems *and* a nursing model. If you cluster data according to

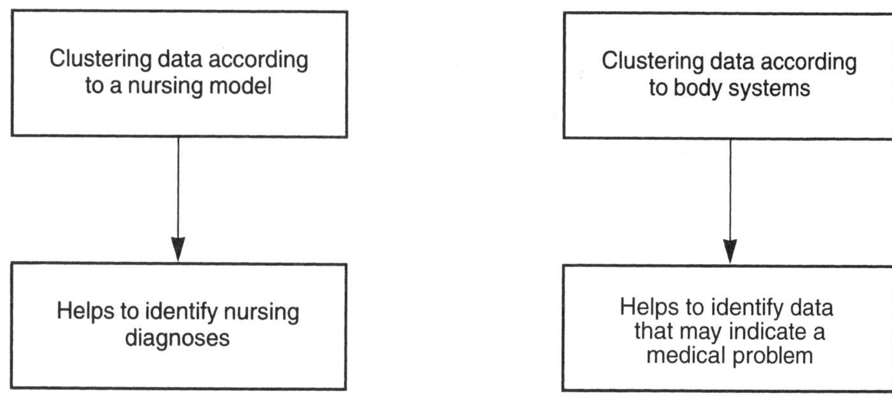
Clustering data according to a nursing model
Helps to identify nursing diagnoses
Clustering data according to body systems
Helps to identify data that may indicate a medical problem

body systems *only,* you're likely to miss key information that helps you identify nursing diagnoses. If you cluster data according to a nursing model *only,* you may group your data in such a way that medical problems may not be so obvious.

Display 2–6 on the next page shows the same data clustered according to human needs, functional health patterns, and body systems. You don't have to memorize these; you'll learn them by using them later on.

Think About It

1. *There are different ways of organizing assessment data.*
2. *How you organize it influences how you see problems.*
3. *Organizing and reorganizing information promotes critical thinking by helping you see different patterns; each organization reveals different aspects of the information, while hiding others.*
4. *Nursing models help you see nursing problems; medical models, or body systems, help you see medical problems.*

DISPLAY 2–5 Clustering Data According to Body Systems

Clustering in this way helps you identify data that should be referred to the physician.

1. Cluster together a brief client profile (vital statistics), including the following:

   Name; age; reason the individual is seeking health care; vital signs; any known medical problems or diagnoses; allergies; or problems with diet

2. Cluster together any data you suspect may be abnormal for any of the following systems:

   Respiratory system
   Cardiovascular system
   Nervous system
   Integumentary system (skin)
   Gastrointestinal system
   Musculoskeletal system
   Genitourinary system

PRACTICE SESSION V

Organizing (Clustering) Data

To complete this session, read pages 57–59. Example responses can be found on page 232.

1. Why is it important to organize data according to both a body systems framework *and* a nursing model? (Three sentences or less.)

2. On a separate piece of paper, cluster the data below according to body systems and according to any holistic nursing model you choose.

Case History

1. Age 36
2. Married, has three small children
3. Occupation: Landscape architect and homemaker
4. Religion: Episcopalian
5. Medical diagnosis: Pneumonia
6. T: 100; P: 100; R: 28; BP: 104/68
7. States she is concerned about how her husband is caring for the children, that it is “tough on him”
8. States she feels weak and tired all the time, but can’t seem to rest because she keeps coughing all the time
9. Appetite poor; is forcing fluids well (1000 mL per shift)
10. Before illness, she smoked a pack of cigarettes a day but has not smoked since hospitalization
11. States she has always been in good health and has never had to be hospitalized (even gave birth at home)
12. States all the tests that have to be done make her nervous; she is worried about getting AIDS from needle sticks
13. Lungs have bilateral rhonchi; she coughs up thick yellow mucus
14. Chest x-ray shows improvement over the past 2 days
15. White blood cell count is elevated at 16,000

3. When you organized the data above, you may have found some categories had no data listed. If this happened to you in the clinical area, what should you do?

DISPLAY 2–6 Examples of the Same Patient Data Organized According to Human Needs, Functional Health Patterns, and Body Systems

Data

1. 21-year-old male
2. Married, no children*
3. Occupation: Firefighter*
4. Ht: 6′1″; Wt: 170 lb
5. T: 98; P: 60; R: 16
6. BP: 110/60
7. Unconscious from head injury
8. Spontaneous respirations
9. Lungs clear
10. History of seizures
11. Foley draining clear urine
12. Wife states he's always constipated
13. Tube feeding via nasogastric tube every 4 hours
14. Extremities rigid
15. Has reddened areas on both elbows
16. Allergic to penicillin
17. Wife states she feels as though she is falling apart*
18. Wife states that before the accident, he took pride in being physically fit*
19. Wife states that they were considering converting to Catholicism before the accident*

Data Organization by Gordon's Functional Health Patterns

- ✓ Health-perception–health-management pattern: 10, 18
- ✓ Nutritional–metabolic pattern: 4, 5, 6, 8, 9, 11, 13, 15, 16
- ✓ Elimination pattern: 11, 12, 13, 15
- ✓ Activity–exercise pattern: 5, 8, 9, 14
- ✓ Cognitive–perceptual pattern: 7
- ✓ Sleep–rest pattern: 7
- ✓ Self-perception–self-concept pattern: 18
- ✓ Role–relationship pattern: 1, 2, 3
- ✓ Sexuality–reproductive pattern: 2
- ✓ Coping–stress-tolerance pattern: 17
- ✓ Value–belief pattern: 19

(continued)

DISPLAY 2-6 Examples of the Same Patient Data Organized According to Human Needs, Functional Health Patterns, and Body Systems (Continued)

Data Organization by Maslow's Needs

- ✓ Physical: 1, 4, 5, 6, 7, 8, 9, 10, 11, 12, 13, 14, 15, 16, 18
- ✓ Safety and security: 7, 10, 13, 17, 19
- ✓ Love and belonging: 2, 17, 19
- ✓ Self-esteem: 2, 3, 18
- ✓ Self-actualization: 3

Data Organization by Body Systems to Determine What Should Be Referred to the Physician

- ✓ Vital statistics (client profile): 1, 4, 5, 6, 7, 10, 16
- ✓ Respiratory system: 8, 9
- ✓ Cardiovascular system: 5, 6, 9
- ✓ Nervous system: 7, 10
- ✓ Musculoskeletal system: 14
- ✓ Gastrointestinal system: 12, 13
- ✓ Genitourinary system: 11
- ✓ Integumentary system: 15

*These data are more likely to be clustered according to a nursing model only, and therefore are not assigned a category under the body systems organization.

Identifying Patterns/Testing First Impressions

After you cluster your data into groups of related information, you begin to get some initial impressions of patterns of human functioning. But you must test these impressions and decide if the patterns really are as they appear. Testing first impressions involves deciding what's relevant, making tentative decisions about what the data may suggest, and focusing assessment to gain more information to fully understand the situations at hand. Like the puzzle analogy, you put some of the puzzle pieces together and you think you know what the picture looks like. However, often those last few key pieces can surprise you with essential details that change the whole picture.

Consider the following example in which a nurse has used a human needs approach and clustered the data under safety and security needs:

- 72-year-old male
- Blind
- States "I hurt myself a lot."
- States "I use a cane to detect objects in front of me."
- Has visible bumps and bruises over arms and on head

The above information suggests that this person has a pattern of injuring himself frequently, perhaps because he's blind. However, there isn't enough data. You need to examine the information, decide what's relevant and irrelevant, and look for reasons why he keeps hurting himself. You may decide the following:

Irrelevant: male

Relevant: elderly, blind, says he's always hurting himself, uses a cane, has bumps and bruises

The above data may support that he injures himself because he's blind. But you need to ask more questions, like, "Does he live alone, or is someone else responsible for his care? Are his injuries really due to blindness?" Perhaps he's falling down because of weakness or dizziness. After all, if he's using the cane correctly, do you think he'd bump himself all the time? These questions that come to mind when identifying patterns guide you to collect additional information to test initial impressions and describe the problems more clearly. For example, with the man above, you might use probing questions to clarify how and why he keeps hurting himself. You may find that he's hurting himself because he's fainting, doesn't use the cane properly, is a victim of abuse, has a low platelet count, or takes anticoagulants.

To focus your assessment on testing first impressions and gaining key pieces of information about patterns of health or illness, keep the following critical thinking principles in mind:

1. **Determine what's relevant and irrelevant:** Ask yourself what *relevant* information might be missing.
2. **Remember cause and effect:** Find out why or how the pattern came to be (ie, look for contributing factors).

Reporting and Recording

The final phase of *Assessment* is reporting and recording. Reporting abnormal data in a timely fashion expedites diagnosis and treatment of urgent problems. Recording data in a timely fashion helps promote:

1. **Continuity:** No one can read your notes when they're in your pocket.
2. **Accuracy:** Your notes are more likely to be accurate and complete when your memory is fresh.
3. **Critical thinking:** Writing information down and then evaluating it to interpret what it means and what might be missing is a key strategy that can enhance your ability to think critically.

Reporting significant findings may take priority over recording comprehensive assessment data. For example, if you take someone's vital signs and find a temperature of 104°F, you report the vital signs immediately before taking the time to record the entire data base.

Whereas Chapter 5 discusses reporting and recording during *Implementation*, this section focuses on deciding what to report and record after performing an *initial* comprehensive data base assessment.

Deciding What to Report

Many beginning nurses have trouble deciding what to report. Until you gain enough experience to be confident in determining what data might be significant of an impending problem, follow this rule:

RULE ➧ Report anything you *suspect* might be abnormal.

Think About It

Reporting anything you suspect might be abnormal to your instructor, preceptor, or supervisor accomplishes three things:

1. *It promotes early diagnosis even if you don't have the knowledge to diagnose the problem yourself.*
2. *It keeps others who are accountable for your patient's well-being informed.*
3. *It helps you learn. Often you receive help determining whether the information is significant.*

Deciding What's Abnormal

There are many factors to consider when deciding what's abnormal (eg, age, disease process, culture, stress tolerance). If your knowledge is so limited that you're not certain what's abnormal, be sure that you work with a more experienced nurse (or instructor). To be safe, ask him or her to review your assessment data until you become more comfortable with identifying abnormalities.

Review Display 2–7, which lists key questions to ask to decide what's normal and abnormal, then consider the following two rules.

RULE 1 ➧ To decide if something is abnormal, compare the information with accepted standards for normalcy; if the information isn't within the limits for normal, it's abnormal. For example, if you're caring for an adult and find a resting pulse of 110 beats per minute, you'd suspect this is abnormal because a normal resting pulse range is 60 to 100 beats per minute.

DISPLAY 2-7 Questions to Ask to Determine What's Normal and What's Abnormal

Ask the Person

- Would you say this is normal or abnormal for you?
- What would you describe as normal for you?

Ask Yourself

- What's accepted as normal for someone who's this person's age? Physical stature? Culture? Developmental status?
- What's accepted as normal for someone who has:
  This disease process?
  This person's beliefs or cultural background?
  This occupation, this socioeconomic level, this lifestyle?
- If I compare the data I've collected with the data gathered on admission (baseline data) or the data gathered in the past 24 to 48 hours, are there changes that reflect increasing problems?
- Are there too many slightly abnormal factors that, when put together, signify an overall picture of abnormality?
- Is what the individual accepts as normal detrimental to his health?

RULE 2 Normal limits may vary from person to person and situation to situation. For example, a pulse of 110 beats per minute may be normal for a child or for someone who's anxious, but abnormal for a sleeping adult who usually has a resting pulse of 56 beats per minute.

The following guidelines can help you make decisions about reporting assessment findings.

Guidelines: Reporting Significant Findings

General Guidelines

- If you find yourself thinking, "I'm not sure if there's anything abnormal here I need to report," you probably don't have enough knowledge to make this decision and need to get help. Consult your instructor, a more experienced nurse, or a reliable text.
- Report abnormal findings as soon as possible. This prevents you from forgetting and may expedite problem identification.
- Before reporting, take a moment to be sure you have all the necessary information readily at hand (eg, patient's name, room number, vital signs, laboratory studies, intake and output, medication record). In emergencies, this may not be possible; instead, ask another nurse to contact the appropriate professional (nurse, physician) while you continue to gather your information.

- If you're nervous about giving the report, jot down the facts in order of importance, then read your list.
- Give precise information. State the facts rather than how you *interpret* the facts. This allows the other professionals to come to their own conclusions without being influenced by your interpretation of the facts.

EXAMPLE

Right: Mrs. Blakely is complaining of a right frontal headache. She received two Tylenol an hour ago, but she's still restless and says she has no relief. Her vital signs and neurologic status are stable.
Wrong: Mrs. Blakely isn't doing well. I think she has a migraine because she already got Tylenol and she's not any better.

- If the person you're talking to doesn't seem to understand the problem after hearing the facts, then state your interpretation of the data (eg, "I'm concerned that she has a migraine and needs something stronger than Tylenol for relief.").
- Chart the time you made the report, the name of the person you notified, and any actions taken on the data base or nurses' notes (eg, "Notified L. Ballard, RN. She assessed the patient and will notify Dr. Sophocles."). Documenting what you reported and to whom you reported lets others know: 1) You observed something you felt was significant enough that someone with more knowledge and authority should be notified. 2) Who is aware of the information (and, therefore, whether anyone else needs to be notified).

Guidelines for Phone Reports

- Identify yourself by name and position. If you're a student nurse, remember that you aren't allowed to take verbal orders. Ask your instructor to listen on another line and tell the physician she's listening (eg, "This is Ms. Pratt. I'm a student. My instructor, Ms. Rae, is listening on the other line.").
- State the patient's name, diagnosis, and room number, then ask, "Do you know whom I'm talking about?" This gives the person time to focus on the particular patient. It also helps you know how much background information might be needed.
- Double check your interpretation of the conversation (eg, "So you don't want to be notified unless the temperature is above 102°, is that correct?").

PRACTICE SESSION VI

Recognizing Abnormal Data, Deciding What's Relevant, Applying the Principle of Cause and Effect

To complete this session, read pages 61–66. Example responses can be found on page 232.

1. **Practice identifying what's normal and abnormal,** by completing the exercise below.
   Study the objective and subjective data below. In the space to the left, put "N" next to the normal data, "A" next to the abnormal data.
   - **a.** ________ States he usually has a bowel movement every other day.
   - **b.** ________ Temperature of 101°F.
   - **c.** ________ Pulse rate of 72 and regular (adult).
   - **d.** ________ Pulse rate of 150 (adult).
   - **e.** ________ Has hives over entire body.
   - **f.** ________ Infant cries as mother leaves the room.
   - **g.** ________ Patient complains of pain with urination.
   - **h.** ________ Grandmother suddenly does not recognize favorite grandchild.
   - **i.** ________ Grandmother says, "I can see okay as long as I wear my glasses."
   - **j.** ________ Infant cries, pulls at ears, and cannot be consoled by his mother.
2. **Practice looking for relevant information:** Turn to the case history on page 21. Consider what questions you might ask to gain additional relevant information you'd need if you were trying to determine how Mr. Moran cares for himself at home.
3. **Practice determining contributing factors** (applying the principle of cause and effect): For the same case history mentioned above, consider what questions you might ask to gain additional information to help you more fully understand factors that might be contributing to, or causing, Mr. Moran's breathing problems.

Deciding What to Record

If you think information is significant enough to report, most likely it's significant enough to record. In fact, a good rule of thumb is *record anything you report.*

How and what you chart is extremely important for the patient's sake and your own protection against malpractice suits. Lawyers consistently stress the following rule:

RULE ➧

> Be sure you follow each facility's policies and procedures for recording the data base. Policies and procedures vary from one facility to another, but you must follow them closely. They're designed to guide you to create a complete data base that provides legal documentation of accepted standards of care.

The following guidelines can help you form good charting habits.

Guidelines: Recording the Nursing Data Base

(Additional guidelines for charting during *Implementation* are on page 165).

- **Use ink and write or print legibly, even when pressed for time.** Your notes are useless to others if they can't be understood, and they'll be useless to you if you're asked 5 years later in a court of law to recall what happened at a given time. Sloppy or illegible notes can also work against you in court; it's easy for a jury to interpret sloppy handwriting as sloppy care.
- **Complete the data base as soon as you can.** Late charting may lead to omissions and errors that can later be interpreted as care that was substandard. If, for some reason, you have to leave the unit before completing the data base, make sure the most important information (eg, vital signs, allergies, medications) is charted before you leave.
- **Chart objectively without making value judgments;** record subjective data by using direct quotes.

EXAMPLE

Right: States, "I don't go to church."
Wrong: Not religious.

- **Avoid terms that have a negative connotation** (eg, "drunk," "disagreeable"). In court they may convey a negative attitude on your part.
- **Keep all information confidential.** In addition to inaccurate or unrecorded information, breach of confidentiality is also a common reason for malpractice suits.
- **Keep it short;** record the facts and be specific about the problems at hand.

EXAMPLE

Right: Breath sounds diminished at left lower base. Complains of "piercing pain" with inspiration at the lower left base. Respirations 32, pulse 110, BP 130/90.
Wrong: Seems to be having breathing problems. Also complains of chest pain.

- **If you make an inference, support it with evidence.**

EXAMPLE

Right: Seems upset. When questioned, he states he's "fine" and that he's "not upset," but he doesn't make eye contact, uses only one-word answers, and states he doesn't "feel like talking."
Wrong: Seems upset about something.

- **If you make a mistake, correct it without covering up the original words.** Instead, draw a line through the original words, write "error" and enter your initials. Never alter a chart without following this procedure; it may imply intent to cover up the facts, which is considered malpractice.
- **If the patient chooses not to answer a question, record "chooses not to answer."** If you gain information from significant others that you think you should record, list the name and relationship of the person to the patient (eg, "Wife states he's allergic to morphine.").
- **Keep in mind that accreditation visitors, lawyers, and insurance companies examine the data base specifically for evidence of the following:** skilled observation and evaluation with notification of physician if warranted; risks for injury and corresponding safety precautions, educational needs and teaching; discharge planning, need for direct skilled nursing care, and use of appropriate resources (multidisciplinary approaches).

Summary

Assessment—the first step to determining health status—consists of five key activities: collecting data, validating data, organizing (clustering) data, identifying patterns/testing first impressions, reporting and recording data. These activities are designed to help you be accurate, complete, and organized as you prepare for the next step, *Diagnosis*. How you organize your data influences how you see problems. To avoid missing nursing or medical problems, be sure to use *both* a body systems framework and a holistic nursing model to cluster your data. Always report and record abnormal data in a timely fashion. It ensures early detection of patient problems and helps you learn (because you find out what data is significantly abnormal enough to indicate a problem).

Evaluate your knowledge of this chapter. Check to see if you can achieve the objectives on page 28.

Bibliography: See pages 189–191.

CHAPTER 3

Diagnosis

OBJECTIVES

Once you complete this chapter, you should be able to:

- Explain why *Diagnosis* is a pivotal point in the nursing process.
- Compare and contrast the *diagnose and treat* model and the *predict, prevent, and manage* model.
- Address the pros and cons of using critical paths and computer-assisted diagnosis.
- Discuss the legal implications of the term *diagnosis.*
- State your responsibilities in relation to nursing diagnoses, medical diagnoses, and collaborative problems.
- Explain the possible consequences of diagnostic errors.
- Identify resources that can assist you to recognize diagnoses.
- Write diagnostic statements for actual, risk and possible diagnoses.
- Use diagnostic reasoning—including taking specific steps to avoid diagnostic errors—the next time you're in the clinical setting.

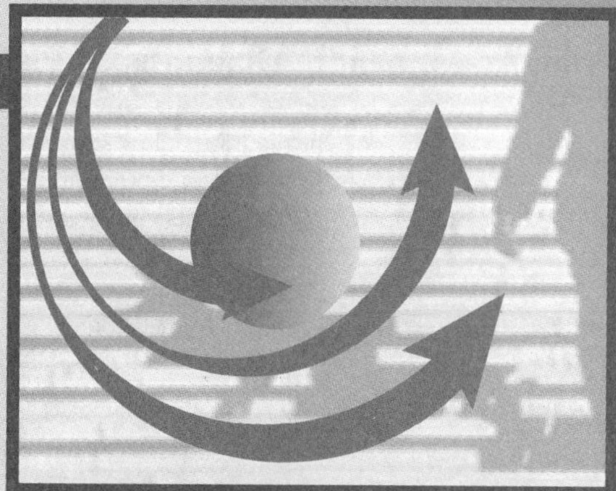

Standard II: ***Diagnosis.*** The nurse analyzes assessment data in determining diagnoses.*

Practice Sessions

- **Practice Session VII:** Nurses' Responsibilities as Diagnosticians/Key Terms Related to Diagnosis/Differentiating Between Nursing Diagnoses and Collaborative Problems
- **Practice Session VIII:** Recognizing Nursing Diagnoses
- **Practice Session IX:** Writing Diagnostic Statements for Nursing Diagnosis
- **Practice Session X:** Predicting Potential Complications
- **Practice Session XI:** Identifying Nursing Diagnoses, Potential Complications, and Strengths

What's in this chapter?

This chapter focuses on the importance of *Diagnosis,* a pivotal step in the nursing process. It addresses how nursing's diagnostic responsibilities are growing, what your responsibilities are in the face of the rapidly changing health care environment, and how to accurately diagnose and record health problems.

*Excerpted from ANA Standards of Clinical Nursing Practice (ANA, 1991).

From Assessment to Diagnosis, A Pivotal Point

The diagram below shows how the activities of *Assessment* lead to what many consider to be a pivotal point in the nursing process: *Diagnosis* (problem identification).* *Diagnosis* is considered a pivotal point for two reasons:

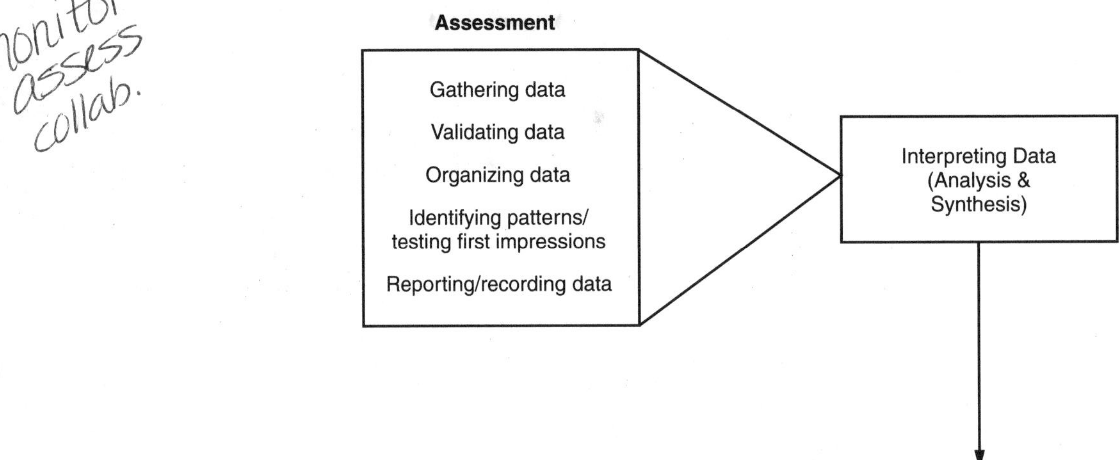

*Although *Diagnosis* involves identifying problems *and* strengths, most people refer to this step as *problem identification.*

1. **The problems you identify during this phase are the basis for the plan of care.** If your problem list is accurate, specific, and complete, your plan will focus on the most important concerns. If it's not, it's likely to result in inefficient, perhaps even dangerous care.
2. **The strengths you identify are invaluable when determining effective nursing interventions.** If you disregard strengths, you may be overlooking one of your most valuable resources: the person requiring care and his or her family and network of support.

Nurses' Growing Responsibilities as Diagnosticians

Laws and standards continue to change to reflect how nursing practice is growing. Some advanced practice nurses are now qualified to diagnose and treat specific medical problems. As a beginning nurse, you're responsible for:

Recognizing health problems
Anticipating complications
Initiating actions to ensure appropriate and timely treatment.

Let's consider five major factors in health care today that impact on your diagnostic role.

1. A shift in thinking about how to approach diagnosis and treatment. Health care delivery has moved from a model of *diagnose and treat* to a model of *predict, prevent, and manage.*
2. The development and refinement of critical pathways (also called *critical paths, clinical pathways, or CareMaps*™*).**
3. Computer-assisted diagnosis.
4. More emphasis on the importance of collaborative (multidisciplinary) practice.
5. Greater awareness that nursing's scope of practice has a flexible boundary that responds to the changing needs of society and its expanding knowledge base (ANA, 1995).

Diagnose and Treat Versus Predict, Prevent, and Manage

So, what's the difference between *diagnose and treat* (DT) and *predict, prevent, and manage* (PPM)?

Diagnose and treat implies that we wait for evidence of problems before beginning treatment. For example, in the past, if people were exposed to *human immunodeficiency virus* (HIV), we monitored them until evidence of the virus appeared in their blood before beginning treatment. Today, using the PPM model, when we know someone has had a significant risk for exposure to HIV, we begin treatment immediately, in hopes of eliminating the virus before it even appears in the blood stream.

DT has a narrow approach that's strong on *treating* problems, but weak on *predicting* the likely course of problems and *preventing and managing* potential complications.

On the other hand, PPM focuses on *early intervention* to minimize problems and prevent or manage their potential complications. This model is based on research findings. We now know the typical course of many health problems—and we know how to alter that course through early intervention.

Using a PPM approach requires you to do two things.

1. **In the presence of known problems,** you predict the *most likely and most dangerous* complications, and take immediate action, to: a) prevent them, and b) to manage them in case they can't be prevented.

EXAMPLE

> As a beginning nurse working in the emergency department, you encounter a woman with a possible heart attack. Knowing you're inexperienced, you quickly report this problem so immediate steps can be taken to minimize the problem and its potential complications (eg, an IV may be inserted, and medications may be given to improve blood flow to the heart and prevent arrhythmias).

*The terms *critical pathways, critical paths, clinical pathways, clinical paths,* and *CareMaps*™ are all used interchangeably.

2. **Whether problems are present or not,** you *look* for evidence of *risk factors* (things that we know may cause problems, such as smoking). If you identify risk factors, you aim to reduce or control them, thereby preventing the problems themselves.

EXAMPLE

> You're performing an assessment and find a teenage boy to be in excellent health. However, you identify that he has risky sexual behaviors. You recognize that this puts the young man at risk for contracting HIV, and you focus on reducing his risk factors for this serious potential problem (eg, you may contact a peer counselor to discuss the need for safe sex).

Using the PPM model requires knowledge of disease process, treatment, and prognosis (the usual course and outcome of injury or disease). Keep in mind that *predict* in the PPM model doesn't mean that a complication *will* happen (eg, my patient has this problem, so he also will have these complications. This would be an assumption). It means you must *anticipate* the possibility of certain complications and be prepared to detect, prevent, and manage them.

Critical Pathways (Clinical Pathways, CareMaps™)

Through research and collaborative practice, most facilities continue to develop and refine critical pathways. Critical pathways are standard plans that predict the day-by-day care required to achieve outcomes for specific health problems within a certain time frame. (See page 240 in the appendix for a critical path.)

When working in facilities that use critical paths, you're often alerted to major diagnoses and predicted care before even meeting the patient. Knowing major diagnoses and predicted care has advantages and disadvantages. It can be helpful in that you quickly learn the usual course of treatment for common problems through repeated experience. It can be a problem in that you may be so influenced by knowing major diagnoses and predicted care in advance, that you may be tempted to take short cuts. For example, it's easy to become complacent (eg, "I already know the problems, so I don't have to worry too much about assessment."). This type of attitude (conscious or unconscious) can make you miss key information that significantly changes the whole picture of patient care. When using critical pathways, keep an open mind and think independently. Always determine your patient's *specific* needs rather than assume he or she "fits" the typical critical path.

Computer-Assisted Diagnosis

Computer-assisted diagnosis can also help or hinder the diagnostic process. Computerized diagnostic programs are designed to help you identify problems. You enter data, and the computer organizes it and suggests diagnoses to consider based on the data. Computers are valuable tools that can expedite problem identification and help you learn. But, you must use them with an active, critical mind, asking yourself questions like, "How does this compare with my patient's situation, down to the last detail?"

It's important to realize the following limitations of computer-assisted diagnosis.

Limitations of Computer-Assisted Diagnosis

Computers:

- Assume data that are entered are true, simply shuffling the information around.
- May not be up to date with minute-to-minute changes in patient status.
- Don't replace humans. Computers have no common sense. Humans analyze and interpret what computers generate, often recognizing obvious errors computers miss.
- Don't relieve you of the responsibility of learning principles and rules of diagnostic reasoning. Knowing these helps you recognize when computers make mistakes.

Think About It

Computers are only as useful as your ability to interpret and analyze the information they generate in context of human situations. For example, not long ago a jet filled with Christmas travelers crashed into a mountain in South America. The computer told the pilots it was flying at a safe altitude, well above the ground. What the computer didn't know was that the pilot made a left turn, pointing straight toward mountains. The pilots relied on the computer's information, neglecting to consider the change in the plane's direction, causing a disaster. As a nurse, you're like the pilot of an airplane, responsible for navigating your patients through the health care maze. Be careful not to rely too much on computer-generated data. Carefully critique the information, in context of the current situation (what's true for patient A, may not be true for patient B, with similar data, but different details).

Multidisciplinary Practice

Increased awareness of the importance of multidisciplinary approaches also impacts on your role as a diagnostician. As a nurse, you must be keenly aware that you don't work in isolation. Many problems require more than nursing resources to be resolved in a timely manner. As you'll see later on in this chapter, you must know when "you're out of your league," so to speak. You have to be able to recognize not only the problems you accept accountability for managing, but also the problems that require management by a physician or APRN.

Society's Changing Needs and Nursing's Expanding Knowledge Base

Nursing's knowledge base continues to expand to meet the changing needs of society. Today's society has a growing elderly population and an increased number of people living longer with chronic illness. We need to know how to help the elderly and those with chronic illness to maximize their independence and sense of well-being in spite of disease. Because of increased emphasis on cost-effective care, people are sent home "quicker and sicker," often requiring nursing care at home. More than ever, nurses are expected to be able to function independently outside the hospital setting, in homes and communities.

Increased awareness of the need for a healthier population also impacts on nurses' diagnostic responsibilities. For example, the government has published Healthy People 2000 (1990), a publication that sets forth goals for a healthy society by the year 2000 (Table 3–1). As a nurse, you're expected to not only recognize problems, but also areas where well people could achieve an even higher level of health.

As society's needs change, nursing continues to expand its knowledge base. For example, the North American Nursing Diagnosis Association (NANDA) continues to develop and refine its list of nursing diagnoses accepted for clinical testing (see inside cover); other researchers are expanding on NANDA's work and examining what nurses do from different perspectives (Display 3–1).

Nursing's knowledge base continues to expand to facilitate nurses' abilities to take on greater diagnostic responsibilities. We have increased responsibilities at almost every level, from staff nurses to APRNs. As the health care environment changes, and as you increase your knowledge and expertise, your diagnostic responsibilities will grow. You'll become increasingly responsible for diagnosing a variety of health problems.

TABLE 3–1 U.S. Public Health Service Priorities for the Year 2000

Goals	Objectives
Health promotion	1. Increase physical activity and fitness.
	2. Improve nutrition.
	3. Reduce use of tobacco.
	4. Reduce alcohol and other drug abuse.
	5. Improve family planning.
	6. Improve mental health and prevent mental disorders
	7. Reduce violent and abusive behavior.
	8. Enhance educational and community-based program
Health protection	9. Reduce unintentional injuries.
	10. Improve occupational safety and health.
	11. Improve environmental health.
	12. Ensure food and drug safety.
	13. Improve oral health.
Preventive services	14. Improve maternal and infant health.
	15. Reduce heart disease and stroke.
	16. Prevent and control cancer.
	17. Reduce diabetes and chronic disabling conditions.
	18. Prevent and control HIV infection.
	19. Reduce sexually transmitted diseases.
	20. Increase immunization and prevent infectious disease.
	21. Expand access and use of clinical preventive services.
Surveillance and data systems	22. Improve surveillance and data systems.

From: *Healthy People 2000: National Health Promotion and Disease Prevention Objectives.* DHHS Publication No. (PHS) 91 Washington, DC: U.S. Government Printing Office.

DISPLAY 3-1 Research Groups Studying What Nurses Do From Different Perspectives (By examining diagnoses, outcomes, and interventions)*

Nursing Diagnosis Extension Classification (NDEC)

- **Purpose:** 1. Describe a collaborative research plan to refine, extend, and classify nursing diagnosis nomenclature.
  2. Improve the comprehensiveness, scope, specificity, clinical usefulness, and clinical testing of the NANDA taxonomy.

Nursing Interventions Classification (NIC)

- **Purpose:** Standardize language describing treatments nurses perform, including direct care and indirect care interventions (direct care interventions include those done through direct interaction with clients, for example, teaching; indirect care interventions include those done away from clients on their behalf, for example obtaining laboratory studies). (Iowa Intervention Project, 1996) (See Appendix C.)

Nursing-Sensitive Outcomes Classification (NOC)

- **Purpose:** 1. Identify, label, validate and classify nursing-sensitive patient outcomes and indicators.
  2. Evaluate the validity and usefulness of the classification in clinical field testing.
  3. Define and test measurement procedures for the outcomes and indicators. (See Appendix D).

---

*Summarized from: Rentz and LaMone (1997).
From Alfaro-LeFevre R. Workshop Handouts © (1997).

So, if you can expect your diagnostic responsibilities to keep changing, how do you know what your responsibilities are *today*? To answer this question, you must first become clearly aware of the definitions and implications of some key terms—terms like *definitive diagnosis, outcome,* and *nurse-prescribed interventions.* These terms, and others essential to learning how to make diagnoses, are listed below in the order you need to learn them (you need to know the first term to understand the next term, and so on).

Definitions and Discussion of Key Terms Related to Diagnosis

Review the following terms, then test your knowledge by completing the practice session on page 84. If you already know these terms, skip to the practice session.

Competency. Having the knowledge and skill to perform an action safely and efficiently.

EXAMPLE

After the first semester of nursing, the student had demonstrated competency giving medications. **Discussion:** You're considered competent to perform an action once you've completed an approved course and passed tests (clinical and theoretical) demonstrating safe practice.

Qualified. Having the competency and authority to perform an action.

EXAMPLE

Although you know you're competent to give IV medications in one hospital, when you go to another hospital, you check policies to determine whether you still have the authority to do so before you can consider yourself qualified to give IV medications. **Discussion:** Authority to perform assessments and make diagnoses is derived from the following: laws, licensure, certification; national, state, and community standards; institutional standards, policies, procedures, and protocols; and other health care professionals (eg, instructors, supervisors, APRNs, physicians).

Nursing Domain. Activities and actions a nurse is legally qualified to perform.

EXAMPLE

Inserting a nasogastric tube prescribed by a physician is in the nursing domain so long as the nurse is qualified to do so. **Discussion:** The nursing domain includes activities that nurses perform independently (eg, monitoring function of a nasogastric tube) and activities that nurses perform when delegated by a physician or APRN (eg, inserting a nasogastric tube). As you progress with your education and clinical experience, your nursing domain will include a wider range of activities. You're responsible for maintaining competency within your practice domain.

Medical Domain. Activities and actions a physician is legally qualified to perform.

EXAMPLE

Performing surgery is in the medical domain so long as it's allowed by law and the physician is qualified to do so. **Discussion:** Some expert nurses now perform some actions (eg, pelvic examinations, removing invasive lines) that used to belong exclusively to the medical domain. When nurses take on responsibility for actions that used to belong only to the medical domain, the actions must be approved by their state board of nursing.

Accountable. Being responsible and answerable for something.

EXAMPLE

If you perform an assessment, and you miss problems, you're *accountable* for what happens (eg, if you miss an area of skin redness, and the area becomes ulcerated because of lack of treatment, you're accountable).

Definitive Interventions. The most specific treatment required to prevent, resolve, or control a health problem.

EXAMPLE

If a patient has *bacterial pneumonia,* you might encourage fluids, assist with coughing, and administer oxygen. However, if you don't have the definitive intervention of giving an antibiotic that's effective against that specific bacteria, you're highly unlikely to get a cure.

Physician-Prescribed (or Delegated) Intervention. An action ordered by a physician for a nurse or another health care professional to perform (Carpenito, 1997b).

EXAMPLE

"Give two units of blood now".

Nurse-Prescribed Intervention. An action a nurse may legally order or initiate independently (Carpenito, 1997b).

EXAMPLE

"Turn patient every 2 hours." **Discussion:** As your qualifications and responsibilities to diagnose grow, so will your authority to prescribe. For example, as we said earlier, some APRNs have authority to prescribe medications, which used to be a physician-prescribed intervention only.

Outcome. The result of prescribed interventions. Usually refers to the *desired result* of interventions (ie, that the problem is prevented, resolved, or controlled) and includes a specific time frame for when the outcome is expected to be achieved.

EXAMPLE

"By three days after surgery, the person who has had a total knee replacement will have stable vital signs, will have no signs of infection, and will be ready to be discharged to a rehabilitation facility."

Judgment. An opinion that's made after analyzing and synthesizing (putting together) information.

EXAMPLE

The nurse was asked, "Based on your professional judgment, what do you think the problem is?"

Diagnose. To make a judgment and identify a problem or strength based on evidence from an assessment.

EXAMPLE

After performing an assessment, the nurse diagnosed *Risk for Aspiration related to decreased level of consciousness and poor cough reflex.*

Diagnosis. In addition, referring to the second step of the nursing process, *diagnosis* can mean two things:

1. The *process* of analyzing data and putting related cues together to make judgments about health status.

EXAMPLE

> The skill of diagnosis is learned through education, practice, experience, and application of critical thinking principles.

2. The *judgment* that's made after the diagnostic process is completed.

EXAMPLE

> **Example of specific diagnosis:** *Ineffective Breathing Pattern related to pain from the right chest incision.* **Example of a less specific diagnosis:** This woman has some type of problem with sexuality; she loves her husband but seems to be having trouble expressing her love physically. **Discussion:** When a diagnosis is very specific, it's easier to identify very specific interventions. There's an important concept to remember about the legal use of the word diagnosis: it implies that there's a situation or problem requiring appropriate qualified treatment. This means if you identify a problem, you must consider whether you're *qualified* to treat it and willing to *accept responsibility* for treating it. If you're not, you're responsible for acquiring qualified help.

Definitive Diagnosis. The most specific, most correct diagnosis.

EXAMPLE

> If you identify signs and symptoms you suspect indicate a myocardial infarction, you begin giving oxygen, take vital signs, and immediately call the physician so a *definitive diagnosis* can be made.

Life Processes. Events or changes that occur during one's lifetime (eg, growing up, aging, maturing, becoming a parent, moving, separations, losses).

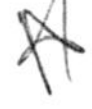

Nursing Diagnosis. A clinical judgment about an individual, family, or community response to actual or potential health problems and life processes. Nursing diagnoses provide the basis for selection of nursing interventions to achieve outcomes for which the nurse is accountable (NANDA, 1994). Nursing diagnoses are often called *human responses* because we, as nurses, focus on how people *are responding* to changes in health or life circumstances. For example, how they're responding to illness or to becoming a parent.

EXAMPLE

> *Risk for Injury related to poor balance.* **Discussion:** The quick reference section beginning on page 193 provides information on each of the nursing diagnoses accepted for clinical testing. However, you don't have to know all the diagnoses. Some diagnoses are in the early stages of development—some you'll never use. When first learning about nursing diagnoses, focus on the ones most commonly used. For example, Display 3–2 lists the diagnoses most commonly used in rehabilitation nursing.

DISPLAY 3–2 Diagnoses: Commonly Used in Rehabilitation Nursing

Risk for Injury
Impaired Swallowing
Pressure Ulcer
Reflex Incontinence
Urinary Retention
Colonic Constipation
Feeding Self-Care Deficit
Bathing or Hygiene Self-Care Deficit
Dressing and Grooming Self-Care Deficit
Toileting Self-Care Deficit
Impaired Physical Mobility
Activity Intolerance
Knowledge Deficit
Pain
Impaired Thought Processes
Body Image Disturbance
Impaired Verbal Communication
Caregiver Role Strain
Ineffective Individual Coping
Ineffective Family Coping
Risk for Disuse Syndrome

Source: American Association of Rehabilitation Nurses.

Think About It

Not all of the nursing diagnoses on NANDA's list are clinically useful to all nurses. The best way to begin to learn which are the most useful diagnoses is to learn them in clusters of diagnoses related to each course. For example, review your fundamentals text or ask your fundamentals instructor about nursing diagnoses you should know as a beginning student, then do the same for maternal child nursing, and so forth. Doing this helps you learn the most common diagnoses first and helps you remember because you learn in a way that's relevant to each clinical specialty. It also saves you time. You don't expect yourself to learn from a long list of medical diagnoses, and you shouldn't try to do this learning nursing diagnoses.

Collaborative Problem. Certain physiologic complications that nurses monitor to detect onset or change in status (Carpenito, 1997). Display 3–3 and the inside cover of this book list common potential complications. Table 3–2 compares the terms *nursing diagnoses* and *collaborative problem.* Figure 3–1 (p. 84) gives a key question to ask yourself to decide whether you've identified a nursing diagnosis or a collaborative problem. **Discussion:** Just because you're a nurse doesn't mean that nursing diagnoses are more important than collaborative problems. The *severity of the problem* is what will help you decide which are your most important concerns right now. As nursing knowledge, expertise, and authority grow, some problems now labeled *collaborative problems* may be considered to be *nursing diagnoses* in the future (because nursing will take on the responsibility for being the primary manager of the problem).

Multidisciplinary Problem. A complex problem requiring ongoing team planning and management by several health care disciplines (eg, nursing, medicine, physical therapy, occupational therapy, and so forth).

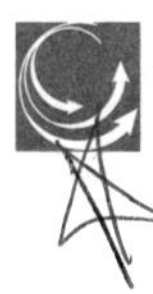

DISPLAY 3-3 Common Potential Complications (More detailed list on inside back cover)

Problem	Potential Complications
Intravenous therapy	Phlebitis Extravasation Fluid overload
Nasogastric suction	Nasogastric tube malfunction Vomiting/aspiration Electrolyte imbalance
Skeletal traction and casts	Poor bone alignment Bleeding Embolus Neurovascular compromise
Medications	Side effects Adverse reaction/allergy Overdosage/toxicity
Foley catheter	Catheter malfunction Infection/bleeding
Chest tubes	Chest tube malfunction Hemo/pneumothorax Bleeding/infection Atelectasis
Surgery or trauma	Atelectasis Bleeding, shock/hypovolemia Electrolyte imbalance Paralytic ileus Oliguria/anuria Fluid overload/congestive heart failure
Head trauma	Bleeding/shock Brain swelling Increased intracranial pressure Coma/respiratory depression

EXAMPLE

Returning a child who has had a severe head injury to school. **Discussion:** In the clinical setting, you may hear the terms *collaborative problems* and *multidisciplinary problems* used interchangeably. For our purposes, *collaborative problems* will refer to *potential complications.*

Medical Diagnosis. A problem requiring definitive diagnosis by a qualified physician. Medical diagnoses usually refer to problems with structure or function of body organs or systems (diseases, trauma).

TABLE 3–2 Comparison of Nursing Diagnoses and Collaborative Problems

Nursing Diagnoses	Collaborative Problems
Main Focus	***Main Focus***
Human responses to disease, trauma, or life changes	Potential physiologic complications of disease, trauma, or diagnostic modalities.
Primary Manager of Problem	***Primary Manager of Problem***
Nurse (may use other resources such as physical therapy or physician expertise, but the nurse accepts primary responsibility for monitoring status and allocating resources).	Physician.
Definitive Diagnosis	***Definitive Diagnosis***
Authority to diagnose is within the nursing domain.	Nurse is required to seek physician diagnosis.
Nursing Responsibilities	***Nursing Responsibilities***
1. Early detection of actual and potential problems. 2. Initiation of a comprehensive plan to prevent, correct, or minimize the problems (nurse is the primary manager of the problems).	1. Monitoring to detect and report early signs and symptoms of potential complications. 2. Initiating actions within the nursing domain to prevent or minimize the problems and their potential complications. 3. Implementing physician-prescribed orders.

Source: R. Alfaro-LeFevre workshop handouts © 1996.

EXAMPLE

> Acute myocardial infarction (MI). **Discussion:** As stated earlier, some nurses in advanced practice are now qualified to diagnose and treat some medical diagnoses.

Related Factor. Something known to be *associated with* a specific health problem (eg, *history of frequent falls* is a related factor for *Risk for Injury*).

Risk Factor. Something known to cause, or *contribute to,* a specific problem (eg, *decreased vision* is a related factor for *Risk for Injury*). **Discussion:** The terms *related factor* and *risk factor* are often used interchangeably.

Etiology. Something known to cause a disease. The terms *risk factor* and *etiology* may be used interchangeably

Risk (Potential) Diagnosis. A health problem that may develop if preventive actions aren't taken.

EXAMPLE

> *Risk for Injury related to poor balance and history of frequent falls.* **Discussion:** Risk (potential) diagnoses are made when you identify risk factors for a specific problem, but have *no* actual evidence of the problem.

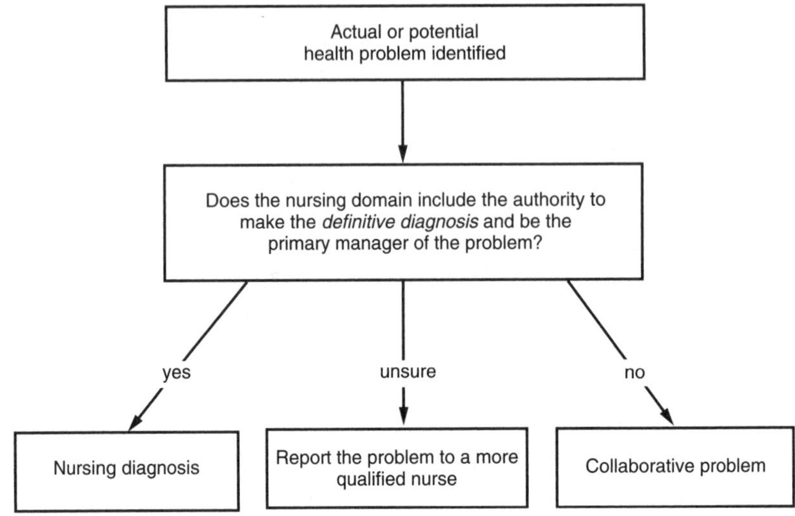

Figure **3–1.** Key question to determine whether you've identified a nursing diagnosis or collaborative problem.

Wellness Diagnosis. A clinical judgment about an individual, family, or community in transition from a specific level of wellness to a higher level of wellness (NANDA, 1994).

EXAMPLE

Potential for Enhanced Parenting. **Discussion:** In most acute care settings, for efficiency's sake, the plan of care addresses only actual and risk (potential) diagnoses, which are considered the most important immediate concerns. In the community and home care, more opportunities are presented to focus on wellness diagnoses.

PRACTICE SESSION VII

Nurses' Responsibilities as Diagnosticians; Key Terms Related to Diagnosis; Differentiating Between Nursing Diagnoses and Collaborative Problems

To complete this session, read pages 72–84. Example responses can be found on page 232.

1. Short answer:

a. How do you know if an action is within your domain of practice?

You may perform an action if qualified to do so.

b. List two key nursing responsibilities related to nursing diagnoses and two related to collaborative problems.

Nsg - Early detection / entiation of plan

Med/Collab - Monitor / Physician orders

2. Check your knowledge of key terms. For each definition below (numbers 1–21), place the letter of the word that best matches the definition. Use each letter only once.

a. diagnose
b. diagnosis
c. collaborative problem
d. medical domain
e. wellness diagnosis
f. definitive diagnosis
g. risk diagnosis
h. accountable
i. competency
j. being qualified
k. life process
l. nursing domain
m. outcome
n. nurse-prescribed intervention
o. physician-prescribed delegated intervention
p. legal implications of using the term *diagnosis*
q. medical diagnosis
r. nursing diagnoses
s. definitive interventions
t. risk (related) factor
u. multidisciplinary problem

1. _____ Something known to contribute to (or be associated with) a specific problem.

2. _____ A health problem for which someone is at risk.

3. _____ The judgment that's made after drawing conclusions about assessment data. May also refer to the skill of analyzing data to make a judgment.

4. _____ To make a judgment and identity and name a problem or strength based on evidence from an assessment.

5. _____ Being responsible and answerable for something.

6. _____ Range of activities and actions that a physician is legally qualified to initiate or prescribe.

7. _____ Range of activities and actions that a nurse is legally qualified to initiate or prescribe.

8. _____ Implies that there's a situation or problem that requires appropriate qualified treatment.

9. _____ Usually refers to the desired or expected result of interventions (ie, the problem is prevented, resolved, or minimized).

10. _____ An action ordered or initiated independently by a nurse.

11. _____ Usually refered to as *human responses*. These provide the basis for selection of nursing interventions to achieve outcomes for which the nurse is accountable.

12. _____ An action ordered by a physician for a nurse or other health care professional to perform.

13. _____ A clinical judgment about an individual, family, or community in transition from a specific level of wellness to a higher level of wellness.

14. _____ Events or changes that occur during one's lifetime (eg, becoming a parent, aging, separations, losses).

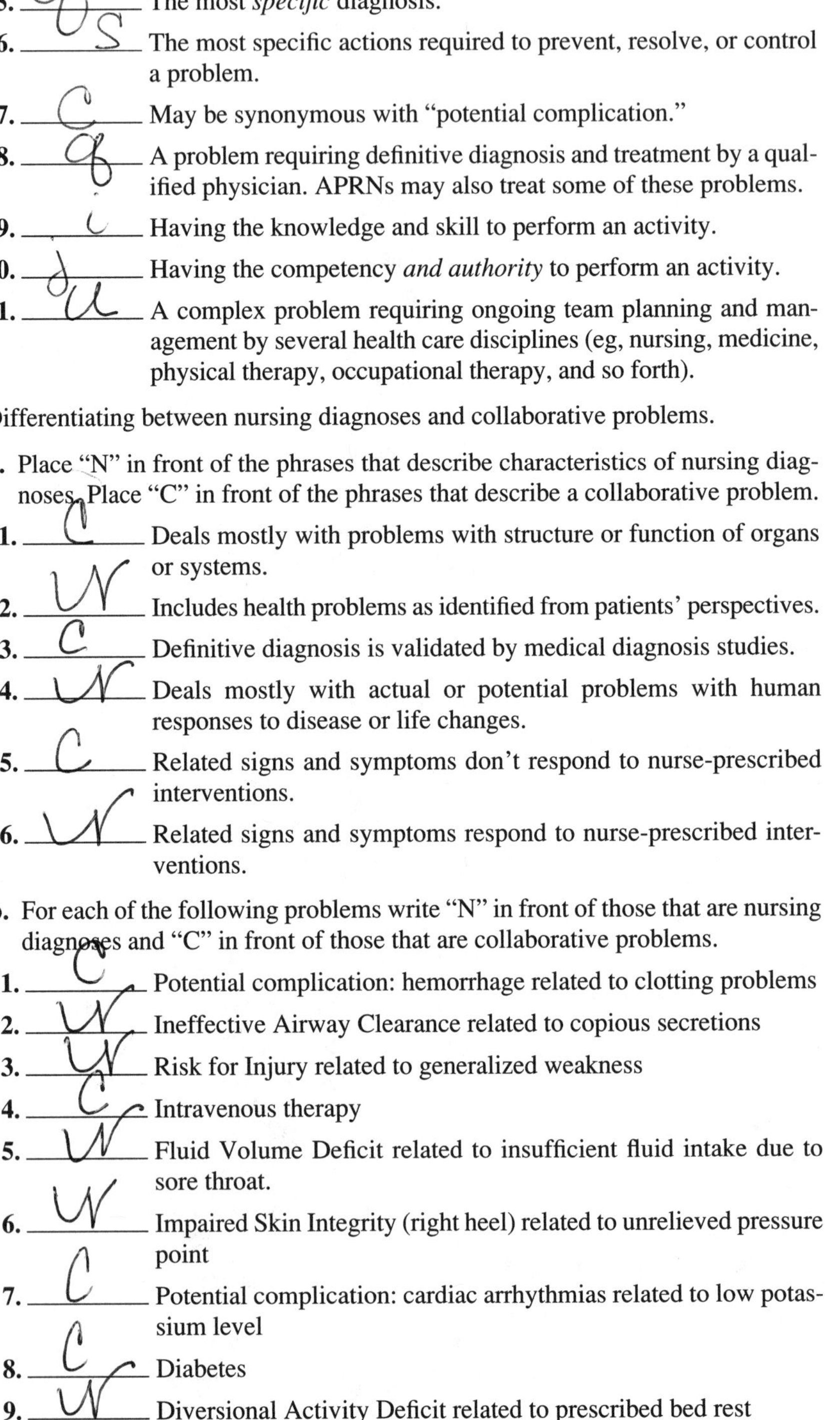

15. ______ The most *specific* diagnosis.

16. ______ The most specific actions required to prevent, resolve, or control a problem.

17. ______ May be synonymous with "potential complication."

18. ______ A problem requiring definitive diagnosis and treatment by a qualified physician. APRNs may also treat some of these problems.

19. ______ Having the knowledge and skill to perform an activity.

20. ______ Having the competency *and authority* to perform an activity.

21. ______ A complex problem requiring ongoing team planning and management by several health care disciplines (eg, nursing, medicine, physical therapy, occupational therapy, and so forth).

3. Differentiating between nursing diagnoses and collaborative problems.

a. Place "N" in front of the phrases that describe characteristics of nursing diagnoses. Place "C" in front of the phrases that describe a collaborative problem.

1. ______ Deals mostly with problems with structure or function of organs or systems.
2. ______ Includes health problems as identified from patients' perspectives.
3. ______ Definitive diagnosis is validated by medical diagnosis studies.
4. ______ Deals mostly with actual or potential problems with human responses to disease or life changes.
5. ______ Related signs and symptoms don't respond to nurse-prescribed interventions.
6. ______ Related signs and symptoms respond to nurse-prescribed interventions.

b. For each of the following problems write "N" in front of those that are nursing diagnoses and "C" in front of those that are collaborative problems.

1. ______ Potential complication: hemorrhage related to clotting problems
2. ______ Ineffective Airway Clearance related to copious secretions
3. ______ Risk for Injury related to generalized weakness
4. ______ Intravenous therapy
5. ______ Fluid Volume Deficit related to insufficient fluid intake due to sore throat.
6. ______ Impaired Skin Integrity (right heel) related to unrelieved pressure point
7. ______ Potential complication: cardiac arrhythmias related to low potassium level
8. ______ Diabetes
9. ______ Diversional Activity Deficit related to prescribed bed rest

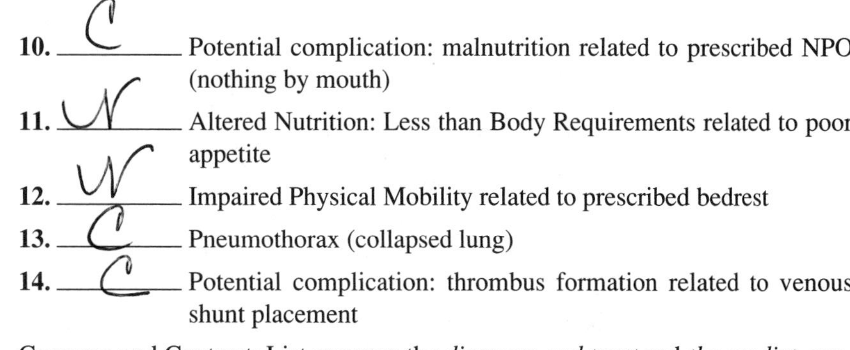

10. ______ Potential complication: malnutrition related to prescribed NPO (nothing by mouth)
11. ______ Altered Nutrition: Less than Body Requirements related to poor appetite
12. ______ Impaired Physical Mobility related to prescribed bedrest
13. ______ Pneumothorax (collapsed lung)
14. ______ Potential complication: thrombus formation related to venous shunt placement

4. Compare and Contrast: List one way the *diagnose and treat* and *the predict, prevent, and manage (PPM)* are the same, and one way that they're different.

Try This On Your Own

Together with at least one other classmate, discuss the implications the statement below has for using critical paths.

Think About It . . .

Critical paths are developed for specific problems, not specific people.

Diagnostic Reasoning: Applying Critical Thinking

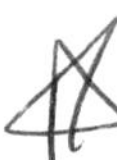

Diagnostic reasoning, or applying critical thinking to problem identification, requires knowledge, skills, and experience. At the big picture level, diagnostic reasoning involves the steps listed in the following box.

Diagnostic Reasoning (Big Picture Level)

- Analyzing cue clusters
- Creating a list of suspected problems
- Ruling out similar diagnoses
- Choosing the most specific diagnostic labels
- Stating the problems and their cause
- Identifying strengths, resources, and areas for improvement

Once you have repeated experiences in various clinical situations, you'll find that diagnostic reasoning becomes almost automatic. However, until then, it's important to be clearly aware of basic principles and rules of diagnostic reasoning. The following principles, rules, and steps are based on sound critical thinking skills like *recognizing assumptions, being systematic and complete,* and *making judgments based on evidence.* They're designed to help you form habits that help you avoid common pitfalls and increase your ability to make accurate diagnoses.

Fundamental Principles and Rules of Diagnostic Reasoning

- **Recognizing diagnoses requires you to be familiar with the diagnoses themselves.** Until you've had repeated experiences with a variety of different health problems, keep references handy. **Rationale:** You can't expect to recognize health problems like *pneumonia* or *Ineffective Airway Clearance* if you don't know what their signs and symptoms look like. By keeping references handy, you begin to recognize problems by comparing your patient's data with the descriptions of the problems listed in the references. You also begin to *remember* what the diagnoses look like because you'll be *using* what you read, rather than simply memorizing words.
- **Keep an open mind.** Avoid tendencies to be overly influenced by past experiences or by information you gain from patient charts or others (eg, you may assess someone whose chart shows a history of chronic back pain related to arthritis and fail to consider that an increase in back pain could signify something else like a kidney problem). **Rationale:** Keeping an open mind prevents you from seeing the problems from a narrow perspective, a common critical thinking error.
- **When you make a diagnosis, back it up with evidence.** Provide the cues (signs, symptoms, risk factors) that led you to make the diagnosis. **Rationale:** Others need to know your evidence so they can evaluate the accuracy of your diagnosis. Cues (signs, symptoms, risk factors) are like "key puzzle pieces"; if you don't have them, you can't complete the puzzle and label the problem. Display 3–4 clarifies the definitions of sign, symptom, defining characteristics, and cues.
- **Although intuition is a valuable tool for problem identification, never make diagnoses on intuition alone—look for evidence to verify your intuition.** Display 3–5 describes how to use intuition safely. **Rationale:** You may intuitively know the diagnosis. However, because diagnosis is based on evidence, you need to validate your intuition.
- **If you miss a problem, mislabel a problem, or identify a problem that isn't there, you've made a diagnostic error,** which may result in inappropriate, perhaps dangerous treatment. **Rationale:** An error in diagnosis is likely to cause an error in treatment. Display 3–6 lists common causes and possible consequences of diagnostic errors.

DISPLAY 3–4 Definitions of Diagnostic Terms

Sign: *Objective data** that have been known to signify a health problem (eg, fever is a sign).
Symptom: *Subjective data** that have been known to signify a health problem (eg, pain is a symptom).
Defining Characteristics: A cluster of signs, symptoms, and risk factors usually present in patients with a specific nursing diagnosis.
Cues: Signs, symptoms, and defining characteristics noted in a patient.

*Often the terms *objective* and *subjective data* are used interchangeably with signs and symptoms. However, technically, objective data include all the data that you observe (normal and abnormal), and subjective data include all the data the patient tells you (normal and abnormal).

DISPLAY 3–5 Using Intuition Safely

- Recognize that while you have no evidence that a problem exists, your intuition is sending up a red flag that says, "There is a problem here; watch this patient closely," or "This patient needs help." Assess closely for existing signs and symptoms that validate the presence of the problem that you suspect. (You should say to the patient, physician, or another nurse, "My intuition tells me that . . ." or "I have the feeling that. . . .")
- If you know that something is wrong, but can't put your finger on any specific problem, increase the frequency and intensity of nursing assessment to monitor closely for early detection of signs and symptoms.
- Before you act on intuition alone, weigh the risks of the possibility of your actions causing harm (either aggravating the situation or creating new problems) against the risk of not acting at all (other than to actively monitor more closely).

- **Just because other nurses have more experience, it doesn't mean they're always right.** When making important decisions, be an independent thinker, ask for rationale, and double-check with reliable resources (references, other qualified professionals). **Rationale:** No one is immune to error; the more experienced nurse may misinterpret your question, or be preoccupied with other duties, and so forth.
- **Know your qualifications and limitations. Rationale:** People have the right to be assessed by a qualified health care professional. Although you may feel that you have the knowledge to perform an assessment and diagnose the problems, you must determine (for your patient's health and your own legal protection) whether you have the authority to do so.

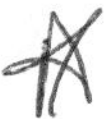

Ten Steps for Diagnosing Health Problems

1. Start by asking the person (and significant others) to identify major problems or concerns. **Rationale:** Often the person requiring care and significant others are the ones best able to identify problems.
2. Be sure you've completed the five phases of assessment, using both a nursing model and body systems model to cluster your data. **Rationale:** Performing a comprehensive assessment and clustering data according to a nursing model and body systems model help you see both nursing and medical problems.
3. Determine normal, altered, at risk, or possible altered functioning (Display 3–7, p. 90), and create a list of suspected actual and potential problems. **Rationale:** This helps reduce the amount of information you're dealing with and helps you begin to focus on problem areas.
4. Consider each suspected problem and look for other signs and symptoms associated with the problem. For example, if you suspect infection because of localized pain and swelling, look for other signs of infection (fever, redness, heat, drainage). **Rationale:** Diagnosis is based on evidence; the more evidence (cues) you have, the more likely you are to be correct.

DISPLAY 3-6 Diagnostic Errors

Causes of Diagnostic Errors

- Overvaluing the probability of one explanation or failing to consider all of the data because of a narrow focus.
  Example: Deciding that anxiety is related to psychological stress, rather than considering whether there might be some physical problem, such as poor oxygenation, causing the anxiety.
- Continuing to *analyze* when you should be *acting* to get help.
  Example: Continuing to see if repositioning and emotional support help a breathing problem, even though they make no difference.
- Failing to recognize personal biases or assumptions.
  Example: Assuming that someone who doesn't bathe daily has a poor self-image.
- Making a diagnosis that's too general (not being specific enough in choosing a diagnostic label to name the problem).
  Example: Using *Altered Patterns of Urinary Elimination* instead of *Stress Incontinence related to weakness of bladder sphincter muscles*.
- Failing to include the correct diagnosis in the initial list of possible problems.
  Example: Listing the problems of *Noncompliance*, but not including the possible problems of *Ineffective Coping* or *Ineffective Management of Therapeutic Regimen*.
- Rushing to get done, either when collecting or analyzing data.
  Example: Rushing through assessment or choosing any diagnosis that's close so you get to report on time, rather than communicating the problem with time to your supervising nurse or the oncoming nurse.

Risks of Diagnostic Errors

When you miss a problem, mislabel a problem, or fail to fully understand a problem, you run the risk of any of the following:

- Initiating interventions that actually aggravate the problems.
- Omitting interventions that are essential to solving the problems.
- Allowing problems to exist or progress without even detecting they are there.
- Initiating interventions that are harmless but wasteful of everyone's time and energy.
- Influencing others that problems exist as described incorrectly.
- Placing yourself in danger of legal liability.

5. Rule in and rule out problems (when you *rule in* a problem, it means you decide it's present; when you *rule out* a problem, it means you decide it's *not* present), looking for flaws in your thinking:
   - What other problems could the cues represent? For example, if a man tells you he's been having increasing episodes of left shoulder pain from an old injury, consider the possibility that this pain could also represent a cardiac problem.
   - What other data could be influencing the status of your suspected problems? For example, you may have *ruled out* the possibility of infection because there is no fever, but when you check all the data you realize acetaminophen has been taken, reducing temperature.

DISPLAY 3-7 Checklist for Identifying Problems

List any history of allergies, disease, surgery, or trauma.

List current medications and intolerance to medications.

	(Circle those that apply)			
Is there a problem with breathing or circulation?	Yes	No	AR*	Pos†
Is there a problem with nutrition or elimination?	Yes	No	AR	Pos
Is there a problem with fluid balance?	Yes	No	AR	Pos
Is there a problem with safety (risk for injury)?	Yes	No	AR	Pos
Is there a problem with rest or exercise?	Yes	No	AR	Pos
Is there a problem with ability to think or perceive environment?	Yes	No	AR	Pos
Is there a problem with communication?	Yes	No	AR	Pos
Is there high risk for infection transmission?	Yes	No	AR	Pos
Is there high risk for impairment of skin integrity?	Yes	No	AR	Pos
Is this admission going to cause difficulties at home?	Yes	No	AR	Pos
Is there a problem with coping or stress?	Yes	No	AR	Pos
Is there a psychological, developmental, or sociocultural problem?	Yes	No	AR	Pos
Is there a problem with personal or religious beliefs?	Yes	No	AR	Pos
Is there a problem with health maintenance at home?	Yes	No	AR	Pos
Is there a problem with role, relationships, or sexuality?	Yes	No	AR	Pos
Does the person have a problem with taking medications?	Yes	No	AR	Pos
Does the patient require teaching?	Yes	No	AR	Pos

*AR At risk for problem (no signs and symptoms present, but risk factors are evident).
†pos: Possible problem (insufficient data, but examiner suspects a problem).

Rationale: Looking for flaws in thinking is a critical thinking principle that helps reduce diagnostic errors.

6. Name the problem(s) by using the label(s) that most closely match assessment cues. For example, if you suspect *Anxiety* or *Fear,* compare the cues with the defining characteristics of *Anxiety* and *Fear*. If the cues are most similar to *Anxiety,* name the problem *Anxiety*. If the cues are most similar to the defining characteristics of *Fear,* label the problem *Fear*. **Rationale:** Diagnosis is based on recognizing when cues are consistent with the signs and symptoms (defining characteristics) of a specific diagnosis.
7. Determine the cause(s) of the problem. **Rationale:** Knowing what's causing the problems helps you determine *specific* interventions. For example, note how *a* below can help you determine interventions, whereas *b* tells you very little.
   a. *Fear related to previous bad experience with general anesthesia*
   b. *Fear*
8. If you identify *risk factors* for a problem but have *no evidence* (no signs and symptoms) of the problem, list it as a Risk (potential) problem (eg, *Risk for Impaired Skin Integrity related to obesity and confinement to bed*). **Rationale:** Identifying potential problems is the key to the *predict, prevent, and manage* model.
9. Share your diagnoses with the person requiring care. **Rationale:** The person has the right to be informed of diagnoses and must be a key player in developing the plan of care.
10. Ask the person if there's anything else that should be listed as a problem. Add these problems to the list. **Rationale:** Whatever the person perceives as a problem *is* a problem.

Three Steps for Diagnosing Strengths

1. Ask the person (and significant others) two questions:

   "Can you tell me some things about yourself that you view as strengths, as healthy aspects?"

   "Can you think of any things that aren't really problems, but you'd like to manage better?"

   Rationale: Answers to these questions help you all to recognize assets and areas that could be improved.
2. Cluster together data that indicate normal or positive functioning. Label these areas as strengths and share them with the person and significant others. For example, you might say, "You've made the decision to seek help, which is a healthy thing to do." **Rationale:** This helps both you and the person requiring care to focus on strengths as well as problems.
3. List the strengths that will assist you in preventing, resolving, or controlling the identified problems. (For examples, see Display 3–8.) **Rationale:** These are the strengths that you use to develop an efficient care plan.

DISPLAY 3-8 Examples of Client Strengths

Physical Strengths

- Is in good health; exercises daily and has excellent cardiac and respiratory reserve
- Is in good nutritional state; eats three balanced meals with few snacks
- Demonstrates physical adaptation; upper torso and arms are powerful (compensating for paraplegia)

Psychological and Personal Strengths

- Demonstrates effective coping; states she copes with chronic pain by using guided imagery
- Is motivated; wants to be independent and healthy
- Is knowledgeable; relates understanding of health care management and available resources
- Demonstrates good problem-solving skills; able to adjust daughter's therapy schedule for optimum results and convenience
- Has strong support systems; mother, brother, church are available for help with child care

Avoiding Diagnostic Errors

None of us is immune to error, but we each can work to develop habits that help us avoid mistakes. Display 3–9 lists questions to ask to evaluate whether you're developing habits that reduce the likelihood of making diagnostic errors.

Considering Lifestyles and Coping Patterns

Because nursing is concerned with medical problems *and* how the problems affect someone's daily life, it's important to consider usual lifestyles and coping patterns. When you're attempting to determine how someone is responding to a change in health status or lifestyle, ask the following questions:

- How does this problem change your life?
- How do you feel you're coping with these changes?
- Tell me how you usually adapt to change.
- Can you think of anything you can do to better adapt?
- What resources (personal, community) might be able to help you cope better?

Determining Causative and Risk (Related) Factors

Ability to identify causative and risk (related) factors depends on your knowledge, experience, and analytical skills. However, there are some questions you can ask to help you identify these factors:

DISPLAY 3-9 Avoiding Diagnostic Errors

Do you:

- Take the time to be sure your data is accurate and complete?
- Look for *evidence* of problems you suspect?
- Recognize your biases and avoid value judgments?
- Consider other problems that the cues might signify?
- Look for flaws in your thinking?
- Identify the cause(s) of the problem(s)?
- Include what the patient sees as problems?
- Choose the most specific diagnostic label(s) that best describes the problem(s)?
- Inform the patient (and significant others) what you see as problems?
- Ask someone to double check you when you're unsure?
- Validate the diagnosis with the client?

- What factors does the person (or significant others) identify as causing or contributing to the problem?
- Are there factors related to developmental age, disease, or changes in lifestyle that may be contributing to the problem?
- Are there cultural, socioeconomic, ethnic, or religious factors that may be contributing to the problem?
- Do your other resources for data collection (eg, medical records, other health care professionals, literature review) identify factors that might be causing or contributing to the problem?

Having discussed the importance of considering usual lifestyles, coping patterns, and causes of problems, let's consider how to recognize specific problems. How do you know when signs and symptoms indicate the presence of a specific nursing diagnosis or collaborative problem? Let's first look at how to recognize diagnoses on NANDA's list, then how to recognize collaborative problems.

NANDA's List of Diagnoses Accepted for Clinical Testing

NANDA continues to develop and refine a list of diagnostic labels that are being studied to determine their usefulness as nursing diagnoses (see Quick-Reference to Nursing Diagnoses section). This list is officially updated every 2 years. Some of the diagnoses on NANDA's list have been only minimally used and studied (eg, *Personal Identity Disturbance*), whereas others have had extensive use and study (eg, *Risk for Injury*).

The box below shows the importance of developing and refining nursing diagnoses.

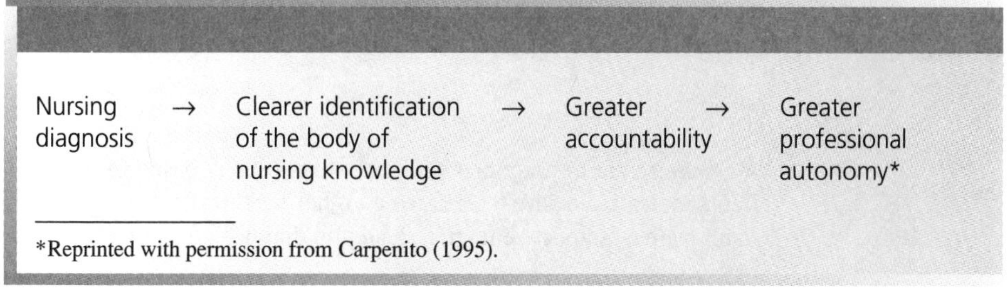

Nursing diagnosis → Clearer identification of the body of nursing knowledge → Greater accountability → Greater professional autonomy*

*Reprinted with permission from Carpenito (1995).

Diagnostic Label Components

Most of the diagnostic labels on NANDA's list have three components:

Title (Label) and Definition: A concise description of the problem.

Defining Characteristics: The cluster of signs and symptoms often associated with the diagnosis. (Risk diagnoses don't list defining characteristics because risk diagnoses are those someone is *at risk for developing*. There are no signs and symptoms evident.)

Related (Risk) Factors: Factors that can cause or contribute to the problem.

To clarify the above, turn to the quick reference section beginning on page 193, which lists all the diagnoses, their defining characteristics, and related factors. Note that, if there are no defining characteristics listed, it's because the diagnosis is a *risk* diagnosis.

Actual, Risk, and Possible Nursing Diagnoses

Recognizing actual, risk, and possible nursing diagnoses requires you to compare the person's assessment data with the definition, defining characteristics, and related

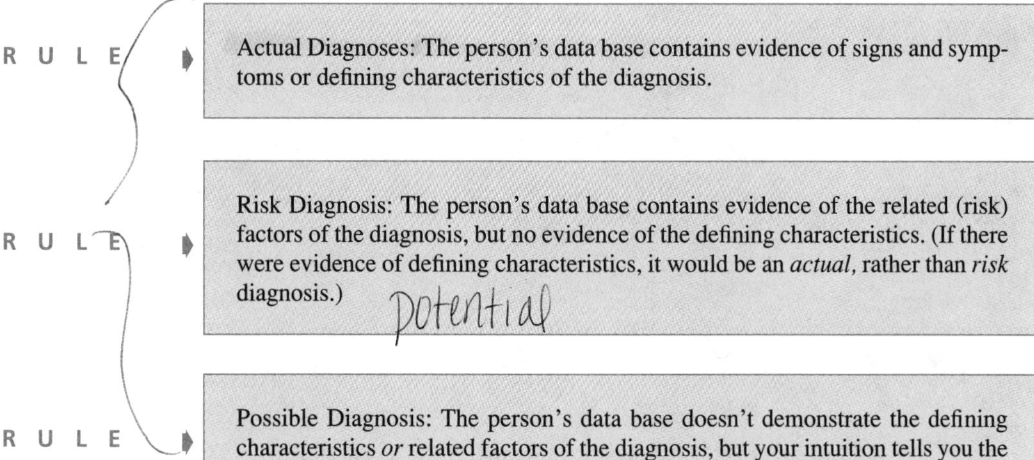

RULE ➧ Actual Diagnoses: The person's data base contains evidence of signs and symptoms or defining characteristics of the diagnosis.

RULE ➧ Risk Diagnosis: The person's data base contains evidence of the related (risk) factors of the diagnosis, but no evidence of the defining characteristics. (If there were evidence of defining characteristics, it would be an *actual*, rather than *risk* diagnosis.)

RULE ➧ Possible Diagnosis: The person's data base doesn't demonstrate the defining characteristics *or* related factors of the diagnosis, but your intuition tells you the diagnosis may be present (eg, *Possible Ineffective Individual Coping*).

(risk) factors of the diagnoses you suspect. Use the rules on p. 95 to help you to identify actual, risk, and possible diagnosis that's on NANDA's list.

Table 3–3 compares the nursing responsibilities for actual, risk, and possible diagnoses.

Wellness Diagnoses

Being able to diagnose wellness diagnoses is based on recognizing when healthy clients indicate a desire to achieve a higher level of functioning in a specific area (eg, "I wish I were a better parent" may lead you diagnose *Potential For Enhanced Parenting*).

Syndrome Diagnoses

There are only two syndrome diagnoses currently on the NANDA list (*Disuse Syndrome* and *Rape Trauma Syndrome*). You use a syndrome diagnosis when the diagnosis is associated with a cluster of other diagnoses. For example, Display 3–10 shows the cluster of diagnoses seen with *Disuse Syndrome,* often seen in bedridden nursing home residents.

TABLE 3–3 Comparison of Actual, Risk, and Possible Nursing Diagnoses

Diagnosis Type	Signs and Symptoms Present?	Etiologic or Contributing Factors Present?	Nursing Responsibilities
Actual Diagnosis	Yes	Yes	Monitor signs and symptoms to determine improvement or deterioration in condition.
Example: *Constipation* poor roughage and fluid intake as evidenced by hard, dry stool.	R/T		Identify interventions to reduce or eliminate the cause of the problem.
Risk Diagnosis	No	Yes	Perform daily focus assessments to determine if signs and symptoms have appeared to change status from risk to actual.
Example: *Risk for Constipation* poor roughage and fluid intake	R/T		Identify interventions to prevent, reduce, or remove risk factors.
Possible Diagnosis	Unsure	Unsure	Gather more data to clarify vague cues and determine if the signs and symptoms or risk factors are actually present.
Example: *Possible Constipation*			

Adapted with permission from Carpenito, L. (1985). Unpublished workshop notes

DISPLAY 3-10 Nursing Diagnoses Associated With Disuse Syndrome

- *Impaired Physical Mobility*
- *Risk for Constipation*
- *Risk for Altered Respiratory Function*
- *Risk for Infection*
- *Risk for Activity Intolerance*
- *Risk for Injury*
- *Risk for Altered Thought Processes*
- *Risk for Body Image Disturbance*
- *Risk for Powerlessness*
- *Risk for Impaired Tissue Integrity*

Nursing Diagnoses Not on NANDA's List

You might identify a problem you think should be considered a nursing diagnosis and not be able to find a label on the list that describes it appropriately. If so, check to make sure you're not making any of the errors listed on page 101 (Guidelines: Avoiding Errors When Writing Diagnostic Statements). If you haven't made any of these errors, describe the problem, its cause, and the evidence that leads you to believe the problem exists (eg, for a young child, you might identify *Bowel Movement Holding related to fear as evidenced by child's statements that she's holding stool because she's afraid of pain, refusal to try to have a bowel movement, and only bowel movement coming at night when the child is asleep.*

PRACTICE SESSION VIII

Recognizing Nursing Diagnoses

To complete this session, read pages 87–97. Example responses can be found on page 233.

This session is designed for you to practice recognizing nursing diagnoses by comparing data with the defining characteristics and related factors of specific diagnoses. Listed below are eight common nursing diagnoses (letters a to h). After the diagnoses are eight different people who have been admitted to the hospital (numbers 1 to 8). For each number, place the letter of the diagnosis that best matches the available patient data. To make the diagnosis: 1) study the data; 2) choose a possible nursing diagnosis from the available choices; 3) look up the diagnosis in the *Nursing Diagnosis Quick Reference Section* starting on page 193, and compare the data with the defining characteristics and related factors for the chosen diagnosis. Each letter should be used only once. To get you started, I have given you the first answer.

a. *Risk for Aspiration*
b. *Activity Intolerance*
c. *Anxiety*
d. *Risk for Impaired Skin Integrity*
e. *Fear*
f. *Ineffective Breathing Pattern*
g. *Ineffective Airway Clearance*
h. *Impaired Skin Integrity*

1. ___b.___ Assessment data for Mrs. Ballard.
Subjective data (SD): Says she feels tired all the time.
Objective data (OD): Lungs clear; becomes short of breath after walking 5 yards; heart rate increases to 130 beats per minute after walking 5 yards; anemic (hemoglobin 7 g).

2. ________ Assessment data for Jim Riley.
SD: States his jaws were wired closed yesterday; complains of nausea.
OD: Jaws wired shut.

3. ________ Assessment data for Charles Lindsay.
SD: States he feels "sort of nervous" but can't pinpoint why.
OD: Restless, glances about, doesn't make good eye contact.

4. ________ Assessment data for Daryl Laird.
SD: States he's very afraid of having to learn to give himself an injection; states he lives alone and is worried something might go wrong when he's alone giving himself an injection.
OD: Doesn't maintain good eye contact: restless.

5. ________ Assessment data for Tim Dydo.
SD: States he's had a cold for 2 weeks and now has pain in lower right rib cage; states he feels like he needs to cough, but finds it too painful.
OD: Respiration 34 per minute; pulse 128 beats per minute; able to cough if rib cage is splinted by me; coughs up thick white mucus.

6. ________ Assessment data for Beth Hendrix.
SD: States she has problems with urinary incontinence.
OD: Wears perineal pad; perineal area red and excoriated.

7. ________ Assessment data for Mary Kay Eipert.
SD: States she's had mild emphysema for 5 years, but now it seems to be getting worse; states she gets out of breath when going up one flight of stairs; says she never learned adaptive breathing techniques.
OD: Expiratory wheezes heard in both lungs; unable to demonstrate pursed-lipped breathing; respiratory rate up to 48 per minute after going up one flight of stairs.

8. ________ Assessment data for Maggie Wolartowski.
SD: Says she's afraid of moving because of pain in her hip.
OD: 92 years old; very thin; had a hip pinning yesterday; skin very dry, no obvious breakdown at present.

Writing Diagnostic Statements for Nursing Diagnoses

Because it's important to be clear and specific, there are accepted ways to write diagnostic statements. Follow the rules below.

Rules for Writing Diagnostic Statements

1. Actual Diagnoses (three-part statement).

   Use PES (Problem + Etiology + Signs and Symptoms) or PRS (Problem + Related (Risk) Factors + Signs and Symptoms) format.

   Use *"related to"* to link the problem and the etiology or related factors. Add *"as evidenced by"* to state the evidence that supports that diagnosis is present.

EXAMPLE

> *Impaired Communication related to language barrier as evidenced by inability to speak or understand English and by use of Spanish.*

2. Risk Nursing Diagnoses (two-part statement).

   Use PE (Problem + Etiology) or PR (Problem + Related (Risk) Factors) format.

   Use *"related to"* to link the potential problem with the related (risk) factors present.

EXAMPLE

> *Risk for Impaired Skin Integrity related to obesity, excessive diaphoresis, and confinement to bed.*

3. Possible Diagnoses (one-part statement). Simply name the possible problem.

EXAMPLE

> *Possible Altered Sexuality Patterns.*

4. For Wellness Diagnoses (one-part statement). Use *"Potential for Enhanced"* before the words that describe the area that is to be improved.

EXAMPLE

> *Potential for Enhanced Parenting.*

5. Syndrome Diagnoses (one-part statement). Simply name the syndrome.

EXAMPLE

> *Rape Trauma Syndrome.*

Making Sure Diagnostic Statements Direct Interventions

Whenever possible, write nursing diagnoses in such a way that they direct nursing interventions. When someone studies your diagnostic statement, it should answer the question, *"What can nurses do about this problem?"* For example, consider the boldface portions of each of the statements below, and note how the first statement directs independent interventions.

Right: Risk for Ineffective Airway Clearance related to **copious thick secretions and difficulty positioning for coughing.**

Wrong: Risk for Ineffective Airway Clearance related to **pneumonia.**

Remember the following rule:

RULE

When writing statements for nursing diagnoses, express them in such a way that the *second part* of the statement (*risk factors*) directs nursing interventions. If this isn't possible, then be sure the *problem* directs nursing interventions. (See the examples below.)

EXAMPLE

Right: *Altered Nutrition: Less Than Body Requirements related to throat discomfort.* Here the related factor (throat discomfort) and the problem (*Altered Nutrition*) can be treated by nurse-prescribed interventions such as providing cool, high-calorie liquids and staying with the person to offer coaching and ensure that the liquids are taken.

Right: *Risk for Aspiration related to wired jaws.* Here, the problem (aspiration) can be prevented by nurse-prescribed interventions, even though the related factor (wired jaws) requires physician-prescribed interventions. Nurse-prescribed interventions would include assisting with clearing of oral secretions, keeping the head of the bed up, teaching how to avoid aspiration, keeping wire cutters at the bedside, and so forth.

Wrong: *Altered Nutrition: Less Than Body Requirements related to NPO (nothing by mouth) status.* Here both the problem and the related factor require physician-prescribed interventions (in the form of IV fluids or gastric tube feedings).

Guidelines: Using Nursing Diagnosis Terminology Correctly

For consistency and clarity, NANDA recommends using the following specific terminology with certain diagnoses:

- Use qualifying or quantifying adjectives to describe the diagnoses when appropriate (Display 3–11).
- If NANDA lists the word *"specify"* in parentheses, it means you should be specific and add the necessary descriptive words to be sure the diagnosis is clear.

EXAMPLE

NANDA lists *Impaired Skin Integrity (specify).* If the skin problem is in the rectal area, write *"rectal"* where NANDA has written *"specify."* Your diagnosis should look like this: *Impaired Skin Integrity (rectal).*

- If you use *Knowledge Deficit* as a diagnosis, don't use "related to." Instead, put a colon after Knowledge Deficit and specify the knowledge that needs to be gained (eg, *Knowledge Deficit: insulin injection technique*).

DISPLAY 3–11 Accepted Qualifying or Quantifying Adjectives

Altered	A change from baseline.
Decreased	Smaller; lessened; diminished; lesser in size, amount, or degree.
Increased	Larger, enlarged, greater in size, amount, or degree.
Impaired	Made worse, weakened, damaged, reduced, deteriorated.
Dysfunctional	Abnormal, impaired, or incomplete functioning.
Ineffective	Not producing the desired effect.
Acute	Severe but of short duration.
Chronic	Lasting a long time, recurring, habitual, constant.
Intermittent	Stopping and starting again at intervals, periodic, cyclic.

Adapted from NANDA (1994).

The following guidelines are presented to help you avoid common errors in writing diagnostic statements.

Guidelines: Avoiding Errors When Writing Diagnostic Statements

- Don't write the diagnostic statement in such a way that it may be legally incriminating.

EXAMPLE

Incorrect: *Risk for Injury related to lack of side rails on bed.*
Correct: *Risk for Injury related to disorientation.*

- Don't "rename" a medical problem to make it sound like a nursing diagnosis.

EXAMPLE

Incorrect: *Alteration in Hemodynamics related to hypovolemia.*
Correct: *hypovolemia.* (This is a medical problem, rather than a nursing diagnosis. Use the correct medical terminology.)

- Don't write a nursing diagnosis based on value judgments.

EXAMPLE

Incorrect: *Spiritual Distress related to atheism as evidenced by statements that she has never believed in God.*
Correct: There may be no diagnosis in this situation. The person may be at peace with her beliefs (not with yours).

- Don't state the nursing diagnosis using medical terminology. Focus on the person's *response* to the medical problems.

DISPLAY 3–12 Checklist for Writing Diagnostic Statements

Is the statement

✓ Based on evidence from the nursing assessment?
✓ Descriptive of both the problem and its cause? Is the problem written before "related to" and the cause written after? For actual diagnoses, have you added "as evidenced by . . ."?
✓ Specific and clear?
✓ Reflective of a problem that nursing has been authorized to manage?
✓ Written with accepted terminology, using NANDA terms for nursing diagnoses unless there's no label on the list to describe the problem?
✓ Free of legally inadvisable and judgmental language?
✓ Written in such a way that there's a high probability that others with the same knowledge and experience agree with the diagnosis?

EXAMPLE

Incorrect: *Mastectomy related to cancer.*
Correct: *Risk for Self-Concept Disturbance related to effects of mastectomy.*

- Don't state two problems at the same time.

EXAMPLE

Incorrect: *Pain and Fear related to diagnostic procedures.*
Correct: *Fear related to unfamiliarity with diagnostic procedures. Pain related to diagnostic procedures.*

Display 3–12 provides a checklist to make sure you've followed the rules for writing diagnostic statements.

PRACTICE SESSION IX

Writing Diagnostic Statements for Nursing Diagnosis

To complete this session, read pages 97–102. Example responses can be found on page 233.

Part I.

1. Practice identifying problems, related factors, and signs and symptoms (PRS): Study the nursing diagnoses below. Circle the problem, underline the cause (etiology, or related factors), and let the signs and symptoms stand as is.
   a. *Urge Incontinence* related to inability to hold large amounts of urine as evidenced by voiding immediately upon realization of need to void.
   b. *Anticipatory Grieving* related to impending death of mother as evidenced by statements of extreme sadness over impending death.
2. Why don't risk diagnoses have signs and symptoms? (One sentence.)

Part II.

The data presented in each clinical situation below matches one of the following diagnoses: *Powerlessness; Altered Nutrition; Less than Body Requirement; Ineffective Airway Clearance*. Study each case, choose the matching diagnosis, and write a three-part diagnostic statement using the PRS (or PES) format.

1. Mr. Stuart demonstrated the following cues (signs and symptoms):
   Subjective (SD): Asks for help clearing secretions; states he can clear airway with help from suction.
   Objective (OD): Copious secretions from tracheostomy tube.
   Nursing Diagnosis:
   Ineffective airway clearance related to copious secretions as evidenced by inability to clear tracheostomy c̄ out suction.
2. Bob demonstrates the following cues (signs and symptoms):
   SD: Reports that he's had no appetite for 2 weeks because of depression.
   OD: Ten-pound weight loss since last visit; 15 lb under recommended weight.
   Nursing Diagnosis: Altered Nutrition; Less than body Requirements related to poor appetite as evidenced by 15 lb below recommended wt.
3. Lilly Johns demonstrates the following cues (signs and symptoms):
   SD: Reports she's depressed and has no control over daily activities.
   OD: She is quadriplegic and has a rigorous schedule of daily physical therapy.
   Nursing Diagnosis:
   Powerlessness related to quadriplegic and rigorous physical therapy as evidenced by depression and feelings of having no choices.

Part III.

The data presented in each clinical situation below matches one of the following diagnoses: *Risk for Ineffective Airway Clearance; Possible Ineffective Individual Coping; Risk for Fluid Volume Deficit; Possible Sexual Dysfunction.* Study each situation, choose the matching.diagnosis, and write a two-part statement, stating the problem and its cause.

1. Mr. Reardon has been confined to bed with casts on both his legs. He seems angry and has stated that he does not want to talk to anyone. You're aware that he's had a fight with his girlfriend.
   Nursing Diagnosis:
   Possible ineffective Individual Coping

2. Mrs. Cappelli has a temperature of 101°F. She sleeps a lot and has a poor appetite. She drinks about 2000 mL a day if you offer frequent fluids and encourage her to drink.

   Nursing Diagnosis:

3. Mr. Rogers has just had his gallbladder removed today under general anesthesia. His nursing assessment form shows that he has smoked a pack of cigarettes a day for the past 20 years. He has a productive cough.

   Nursing Diagnosis:

4. You see Mrs. Jackson in clinic 3 months after a hysterectomy. She states that she feels well physically, but that emotionally she just doesn't feel like herself yet. She states that she gets angry easily, cries a lot, and that she's concerned the hysterectomy is affecting her emotionally and physically.

   Nursing Diagnosis:

Part IV.

Identifying correctly stated nursing diagnoses.

A. Put a "C" in front of each nursing diagnosis that is stated correctly.

1. ________ *Risk for Constipation related to confinement to bed.*
2. ________ *Risk for Injury related to lack of side rails on bed.*
3. ________ *Pain and Anxiety related to surgery.*
4. ________ *Hopelessness related to progressive disease process.*
5. ________ *Spiritual Distress related to atheism.*
6. ________ *Mastectomy related to cancer.*
7. ________ *Altered Skin Integrity (1" blister on heel) related to heel pressure and rubbing on sheets.*
8. ________ *Altered Hemodynamics related to hemorrhage.*
9. ________ *Impaired Physical Mobility related to joint pain as evidenced by reports of pain limiting movement of joints.*
10. ________ *Altered Nutrition: Less than Body Requirements related to being NPO as evidenced by inability to take food by mouth.*

B. For each diagnosis you identified as being incorrect, explain the reason it's incorrect.

Identifying Potential Complications

Remember that *collaborative problems* refer to *potential complications* (PCs). If you're a novice, you may find it difficult to predict and detect PCs. For example, you may examine someone who has chronic respiratory problems and has wheezing, coughing, and shortness of breath even when he's well. It may be difficult for you to know whether these abnormal findings are part of the person's usual pattern of chronic illness or whether the data indicate early signs and symptoms of potential complications.

Your ability to predict and detect PCs will grow as your nursing knowledge expands and you have repeated experiences assessing people with different types of problems. Some knowledge can only be gained by clinical experience (eg, you have to listen to many lungs to clearly know what abnormal breathsounds sound like). Until you acquire this experience, the following rules and guidelines can help you act in your patients' best interest, making sure that PCs are prevented, detected, and managed in a timely fashion.

RULE 1 ➧ Until you feel confident identifying potential complications, report all abnormal data. What may seem like an isolated cue to you may prompt a more experienced person (or someone who knows the person better) to be concerned.

RULE 2 ➧ If you need to write a diagnostic statement for a collaborative problem, focus on the *potential complications* of the problem. Use "PC" (for potential complication), followed by a colon, and list the complications that might occur. For clarity, link the potential complications and the collaborative problem by using "related to." Example: PC: pneumothorax related to fractured ribs.

RULE 3 ➧ **Critical thinking:** Onset of complications is often subtle. Signs and symptoms gradually worsen over a period of time, making changes less obvious. Always compare abnormal data with data charted over the last 24 to 48 hours (sometimes longer). If you see increasingly abnormal signs and symptoms, you may be looking at early signs and symptoms of potential complications. Example: You get a temperature reading of 99.6°F. You compare the reading with temperatures over the past 24 to 48 hours. If it's a new elevation, you may be detecting early complications and know you have to monitor the person more closely.

Guidelines: Identifying Potential Complications

- Look up all medications taken. Consider the likelihood of the patient experiencing side effects, adverse reactions, or effects of drug interactions.
- Read patient records (medical history and physical, nursing history and physical, progress reports, consultations, diagnostic studies). Often medical diagnoses and associated complications are addressed in these records.
- Look up the most common complications associated with the person's medical problems before you begin nursing care (for examples of common potential complications, see inside cover).
- Review critical paths, policies, procedures, protocols, and standards that address your patient's situations (eg, management of chest tubes). These often guide you to assess for specific signs and symptoms you must report to monitor for potential complications.
- Be aware of recent diagnostic or treatment modalities and determine whether there are associated potential complications (eg, thrombi, emboli, and bleeding are potential complications of cardiac catheterization).
- Be sure you determine not only the potential complications, but also the signs and symptoms that indicate onset of the complications. For example, if you suspect pulmonary emboli, determine what signs and symptoms may indicate pulmonary emboli (pain, shortness of breath, anxiety).
- In complex situations, check with a more qualified professional. For example, you might say to an attending physician or a clinical nurse specialist, "There's a lot going on with this patient. Are there any specific signs and symptoms we should be concerned about?"
- If you want to write a diagnostic statement for potential complications, use "PC" (potential complication), followed by a colon, then name the potential complication.

EXAMPLE

PC: pneumothorax

Identifying Problems Requiring a Multidisciplinary Approach

The key question to ask when identifying a need for a multidisciplinary approach is:

Looking at the big picture of this person's situation, is it likely that he/she will be able to reach the desired outcomes in the expected time frame using only nursing expertise for management of care?

If the answer is "no," initiate appropriate referrals. For example, if the outcome for a healthy woman having a hysterectomy is "*will ambulate the first day after surgery,*" you could expect to achieve this outcome using nursing resources alone. However, if the woman has other coexisting problems, for example, difficulty walking due to neuromuscular problems, you might want to consider requesting a physical therapist's involvement with planning and managing ambulation.

PRACTICE SESSION X

Predicting Potential Complications/ Identifying Problems Requiring a Multi-disciplinary Approach

To complete this session, read pages 105–107. Example responses can be found on page 233.

Practice identifying potential complications. Imagine you're looking after someone with each of the collaborative problems below. After the letters **PC** (potential complications), predict the potential complications you'll need to look for. May use inside back cover as a guide

Part I.

1. Intravenous Therapy
PC:

2. Concussion
PC:

3. Myocardial Infarction
PC:

4. Nasogastric Suction
PC:

Part II.

How would you decide if your patient's problems are such that they may require a multidisciplinary approach (ongoing planning and management by a team of health care professionals)? (One to three sentences.)

PRACTICE SESSION XI

Identifying Nursing Diagnoses, Collaborative Problems, and Strengths

To complete this practice session, read pages 105–107.

Study the data given for the following case history. On a separate piece of paper, list the strengths, nursing diagnoses, and collaborative problems that you can identify.

Case History A (Mrs. Goode, 31 years old)

Medical Diagnosis: *cerebral concussion*

Subjective Data

States she has a headache and feels dizzy when she lifts her head off the pillow.
Expressed concern about having her husband look after her two children because "he is not good with them."
States she is afraid of hospitals and needles.
States she has never worked outside the home because her children need her.
States, "I can't stay in bed and use the bedpan as the doctor said."

Objective Data

Age: 31; Ht: 5′8″; Wt: 160 lb
Temperature: 98.4°F
Pulse: 78 and regular
Respirations: 24 and nonlabored
Blood Pressure: 128/72
Moves all extremities with equal strength
Pupils are equally reactive to light
Large bruise over right forehead
Abdomen soft, nontender, obese
Peripheral pulses strong
IV in right arm running at 30 mL/h

Summary

Figure 3–2 provides a visual summary of this chapter, illustrating the diagnostic process. Health care delivery has shifted from a *diagnose and treat* to a *predict, prevent, and manage* model. Nurses' diagnostic responsibilities continue to change and are affected by use of critical pathways, computer-assisted diagnosis, multidisciplinary practice, society's changing needs, and nursing's expanding knowledge base.

Diagnostic reasoning, or applying critical thinking to identifying problems and strengths, requires knowledge, skills, and experience. As your knowledge and clinical expertise grow, your accountability for diagnosis and treatment will also grow. To determine your diagnostic responsibilities, you need a clear understanding of all the terms listed in the practice session on pages 77–84. At the big picture level, diagnostic reasoning involves analyzing cue clusters, creating a list of suspected problems, ruling out similar diagnoses, choosing the most specific diagnostic labels, stating the diagnoses and their causes, and identifying strengths, resources, and areas for improvement.

Statements for actual nursing diagnoses are written using the *PRS* (Problem, Related Factors, Signs and Symptoms) or *PES* (Problem, Etiology, Signs and Symptoms) format. Risk diagnoses use the same format, only the signs and symptoms aren't listed. Wellness diagnoses are one-part statements that use *Potential for Enhanced* as a descriptor. Syndrome diagnoses are one-part statements, simply stating the syndrome. Collaborative problems focus on *potential complications* and are addressed by using PC (see rule #2, page 105). Table 3–2 compares your responsibilities for nursing diagnoses and collaborative problems.

The key question to ask when identifying a need for a multidisciplinary approach is: *Looking at the big picture of this person's situation, is it likely that he/she will be able to reach the desired outcomes in the expected time frame using only nursing expertise for management of care?* If the answer is "no," then initiate appropriate referrals.

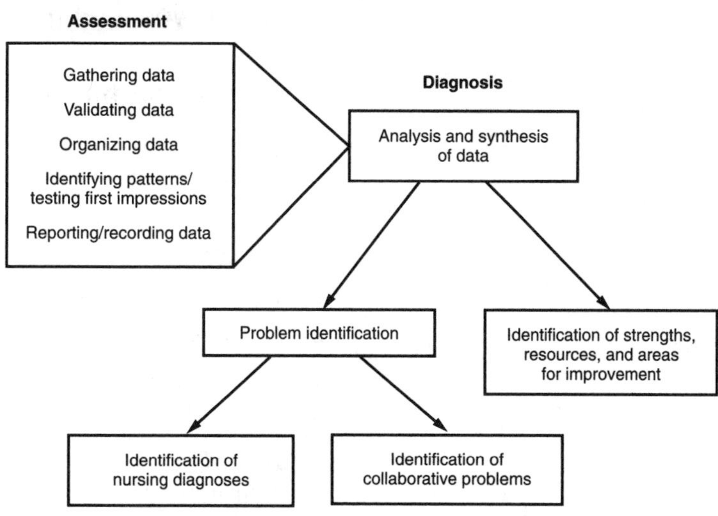

Figure **3–2.** The diagnostic process.

Evaluate your knowledge of this chapter. Check to see if you can achieve the objectives on page 70.

Bibliography: See pages 189–191.

CHAPTER 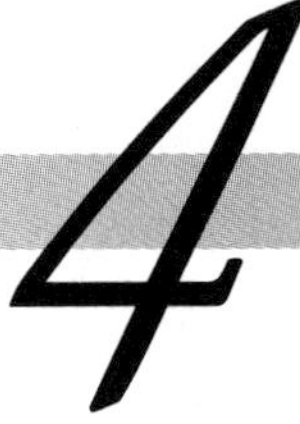

Planning

OBJECTIVES

Once you complete this chapter, you should be able to:

- Explain why every plan of care should have three components (problem list, expected outcomes, interventions).
- Decide how you'll set priorities the next time you're in the clinical setting.
- Name five things that influence priority ratings.
- Give four reasons why specific, measurable outcomes are the key to efficient planning.
- Address the relationship of outcomes to accountability.
- Discuss how to use standards plans (eg, critical paths, guidelines, computerized plans).
- Explain the role of case management in planning efficient care.
- Discuss how to weigh risks and benefits when determining nursing interventions.
- Develop a comprehensive plan of care.

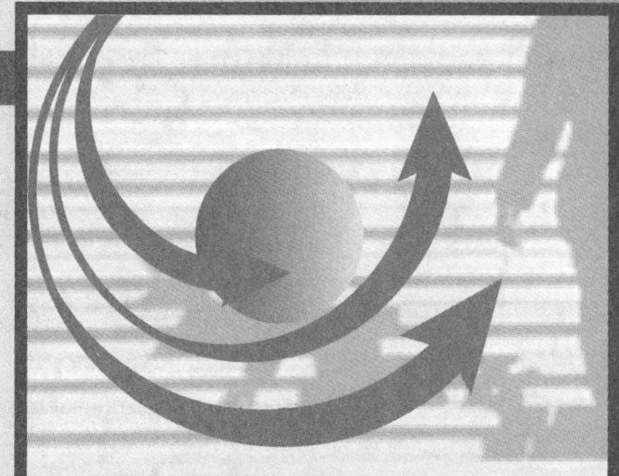

Standard III: ***Outcome Identification.*** The nurse identifies outcomes individualized to the client.*

Standard IV: ***Planning.*** The nurse develops a plan of care that prescribes interventions to attain expected outcomes.*

Practice Sessions

- **Practice Session XII:** Setting Priorities and Applying Standards
- **Practice Session XIII:** Planning Outcome-Based Care
- **Practice Session XIV:** Determining Interventions and Recording Nursing Orders

What's in this chapter?

Emphasizing the importance of outcome-based practice, this chapter provides the how to's of developing and recording an initial plan of care. It guides you through the process of setting priorities and identifying realistic outcomes and interventions. It also addresses your responsibilities for recording a plan of care and using standard plans such as critical pathways and computerized care plans.

*Excerpted from ANA Standards of Clinical Nursing Practice (ANA, 1991).

Planning: Setting Priorities, Establishing Expected Outcomes, and Recording the Plan of Care

This chapter focuses on how to develop an *initial* plan of care. Chapter 5 addresses the *ongoing* planning you do after the plan of care is implemented.

Planning involves the following:

- Setting priorities
- Establishing outcomes
- Determining nursing orders
- Recording the plan of care

Let's first take a look at why care planning rules are so specific, and then address how to develop and record a clear, specific plan that meets the requirements of most health care facilities.

Why Are Rules for Recording the Plan of Care So Specific?

The plan of care serves four main purposes. It

1. Promotes communication between caregivers.
2. Directs care and documentation.
3. Creates a record that can later be used for evaluation, research, and legal reasons.
4. Provides documentation of health care needs for insurance reimbursement purposes.

Different professionals may need to look at the same care plan for different reasons. For example, staff nurses need to be able to determine what care must be given, researchers may need to track specific data, and insurance providers must know what services were required. To ensure that *all key players* in health care delivery have easy access to the information they need, laws and standards mandate that care plans be specific, clear, and consistent.

Major Care Plan Components

There are three major components to the plan of care:

1. **Diagnoses or problems:** What are the problems requiring a recorded plan of care?
2. **Expected (desired) outcomes:** What results do you expect, and by when do you expect you'll see these results?
3. **Interventions:** What's going to be done to achieve the expected outcomes?

Let's look at the first component above—how do you set priorities and decide which problems need to be recorded on the plan of care?

Setting Priorities

Some nurses will tell you setting priorities begins with deciding what problems to deal with first. Others will tell you it begins with identifying discharge outcomes. In a way, they're both right:

- You need to determine urgent problems (eg, those requiring immediate medical attention).
- You need to determine discharge outcomes to decide what must be done first in the big picture of the whole plan.

For example, consider the two discharge outcomes below.

Outcome for Mrs. Matlack: Three days after surgery, Mrs. Matlack will be discharged home, able to demonstrate wound care.

Outcome for Mr. Newsome: Three days after surgery, Mr. Newsome will be discharged to a skilled nursing facility for wound care management.

If you didn't know that Mrs. Matlack would go home and Mr. Newsome would go to a skilled nursing facility, how would you know whether teaching about wound care is a high priority?

Critical Thinking and Setting Priorities

Setting priorities is an essential critical thinking skill that requires you to be able to decide:

1. Which problems need immediate attention and which ones can wait.
2. Which problems are your responsibility and which ones you need to refer to another health care professional.
3. Which problems will be dealt with by using standard plans (eg, critical paths, standards of care).
4. Which problems *aren't* covered by standard plans but must be addressed to ensure a safe hospital stay and timely discharge.

To be able to set priorities, you need to be very familiar with the following principles of setting priorities.

Fundamental Principles of Setting Priorities

- Choose a method of assigning priorities and use it consistently. For example, many nurses use Maslow's Hierarchy of Needs, illustrated in Display 4–1.
- Assign a high priority to problems that are *contributing factors* to other problems. For example, if someone has joint pain and isn't moving well, give the pain a high priority because it's likely to contribute to problems moving.

DISPLAY 4–1 Setting Priorities According to Maslow's Hierarchy of Needs

- ✓ Priority 1: Life-threatening problems and those interfering with physiologic needs (eg, problems with respiration, circulation, nutrition, hydration, elimination, temperature regulation, physical comfort).
- ✓ Priority 2: Problems interfering with safety and security (eg, environmental hazards, fear).
- ✓ Priority 3: Problems interfering with love and belonging (eg, isolation or loss of a loved one).
- ✓ Priority 4: Problems interfering with self-esteem (eg, inability to wash hair, perform normal activities).
- ✓ Priority 5: Problems interfering with the ability to achieve personal goals.

- Your ability to successfully set priorities is influenced by your understanding of:
    - The person's perception of priorities. If the person doesn't agree with your priorities, it's unlikely the plan will succeed.
    - The *whole picture* of problems at hand. For example, if you have someone who is having trouble breathing, normally you'd correct this problem first. However, if in looking at the *whole picture* you note that the person is having trouble breathing because of an anxiety attack, you might decide that resolving the anxiety is the most important problem *right now*.
    - The person's overall health status and expected discharge outcomes. As stated earlier, teaching may have a high priority for someone who's expected to be discharged home, but it may take a lower priority for someone who's expected to be discharged to an extended-care facility (eg, a nursing home).
    - The expected length of stay. For short stays, you must focus on what *must* be done before what's *nice* to do.
    - How standard plans (eg, critical pathways, guidelines, protocols, procedures, standards of care) apply to the person's situation. For definitions of these terms, see Display 4–2.

Suggested Steps for Setting Priorities

Step 1. Ask, "What problems need immediate attention and what could happen if I wait until later to attend to them?" Take immediate appropriate action to initiate treatment as indicated (eg, notify the charge nurse and initiate actions to reduce the problem). **Rationale:** Identifying what could happen if you wait until later to resolve a problem helps determine what must be done. Initiating a call for help expedites treatment for severe problems while you continue to act independently.

Step 2. Identify problems with simple solutions (eg, repositioning) and initiate actions to solve them. **Rationale:** Sometimes simple problems have a big impact on the person's physiologic or psychological status.

DISPLAY 4-2 Definitions of Terms Related to Standards

Note: Although there are varying formal definitions of the following terms, these definitions are designed to be understandable for beginning nursing students.

Critical Pathways or CareMaps™: Standard plans developed to help set daily care priorities, promote timely achievement of outcomes, and reduce length of hospital stays (eg, see page 240).
Guidelines, Protocols, Policies, and Procedures: Documents that delineate how care is to be provided in specific situations.
Standards: Authoritative statements by which the nursing profession describes the responsibilities for which its practitioners are accountable (ANA, 1991). See also guidelines above.
Standard of Care: A document outlining the minimal level of routine care provided for all patients in certain situations (focuses on what will be observed *in the patient* to let you know the care has been given).
Standard Care Plan: A preformulated plan that can be used as a guide to expedite development and documentation of a plan of care.
Standard of Practice: A document outlining what the *nurse will do* in giving care in specific situations. See also guidelines above.
Standard of Professional Performance: Authoritative statements that describe a competent level of behavior in the professional role (see page 21).

Step 3. On a worksheet, develop an initial problem list, identifying the problems and their causes, if known. **Rationale:** This ensures none of the problems are overlooked and helps you get an idea of the big picture of problems (eg, whether one problem might be causing another).

Step 4. Study your problem list and decide what problems will be primarily managed by nursing (nursing diagnoses), what problems are addressed by standard plans, and what problems require multidisciplinary planning. Check whether you have medical orders or facility guidelines to manage medical problems; notify the physician or APRN if you don't. **Rationale:** It's your responsibility to refer problems outside your expertise in a timely manner.

Step 5. Decide which problems *must* be addressed by the plan of care (ie, *which problems must be controlled or resolved in order to progress to achieving the major outcomes of care*). **Rationale:** Records must communicate nurses' awareness of, and responsiveness to, all care priorities. Some problems may not need to be recorded on the care plan because they're addressed in other parts of the record (eg, Foley catheter care is usually addressed in policy and procedure manuals).

Step 6. Determine how each problem will be managed (eg, Medical orders? Following protocols? Nurse-developed individualized plan?). **Rationale:** Policies vary from one facility to another; you must identify where to record a problem and how to manage it according to each particular facility's policies. Figure 4–1 presents a sample worksheet for a problem list showing how a nurse has decided to address care management.

Problem	Care Management Plan
HRF Impaired Skin Integrity R/T Bedrest	✓ Unit protocol
PC: Compromised Respiratory Function R/T Chest Tubes	✓ Chest tube policy & physician's orders
Decisional Conflict (whether to have surgery or wait 2 weeks)	✓ Add to nursing care plan
Spiritual Distress	✓ Refer to Chaplain

Figure **4–1.** Sample worksheet used to develop problem list and care management.

Think About It

When making decisions about setting priorities, it's helpful to ask yourself negative questions. *Negative questions begin with, "What could happen if I* **don't** *. . . ?" For example, "What could happen to this person if I* **don't** *address this problem on the plan of care?" or "What could happen if I* **don't** *report this problem?" Asking yourself these types of questions helps you focus on what's most important. If the answer is "not much can happen," you know the problem has a low priority. If the answer causes you concern, then you know the problem has a high priority.*

Applying Nursing Standards

There are guidelines and standards that you must apply to developing the plan. These standards are determined by the following:

- **The Law:** Your state's nurse practice act delineates the scope of nursing practice.
- **The American Nurses Association** (ANA) and **Canadian Nurses Association (CNA).**
- **Specialty Professional Organizations,** such as the Emergency Nurses Association and the Critical Care Nurses Association, develop standards for specialty practice.
- **The Joint Commission of Accreditation of Healthcare Organizations (JCAHO):** This powerful accrediting body has developed detailed standards that must be followed to keep accreditation.
- **The Agency for Health Care Policy and Research (AHCPR):** This organization develops, reviews, and updates clinical guidelines to aid health care providers prevent, diagnose, and manage certain common clinical conditions (Display 4–3).
- **The Facility Where You Work:** Each facility usually develops its own unique set of standards (standards of care, guidelines, policies, procedures, critical pathways, standard care plans, and so forth) that reflect how nursing care should be delivered in a specific situation (Display 4–4 shows an example).

Planning Outcome-Based (Client-Centered) Care

Effective health care delivery requires us to focus on client *results,* which are stated as *client-centered outcomes:* What exactly do we expect the client to accomplish, and by when do we expect it will be accomplished?

DISPLAY 4-3 Agency for Health Care Policy and Research (AHCPR) Practice Guidelines

Acute and chronic incontinence
Acute low back problems
Acute pain
Benign prostatic hypertrophy
Cancer screening
Cardiac rehabilitation
Cataracts in adults
Colorectal cancer
Heart failure
Managing cancer pain
Depression in primary care
Otitis media with effusion
Post stroke rehabilitation
Pressure ulcer treatment
Quality determinants of mammography
Unstable angina
Screening for Alzheimer's disease
Sickle cell disease
Smoking cessation

DISPLAY 4-4 Standard of Nursing Care for Patients Admitted for Abdominal Surgery

Overall Goal: The individual will experience a safe, comfortable recovery from abdominal surgery with prevention of, and early detection and treatment of, possible complications as evidenced by the following:

1. Before and after surgery, the patient or caregiver will be able to:
    - explain the type of surgery to be done in his/her own words
    - describe the preoperative and postoperative therapeutic plan of care and its rationale
    - relate the expected length of recuperation
    - voice concerns, anxieties, or fears and receive appropriate counseling/interventions as necessary
    - participate in measures to aid recovery and prevent complications
2. During the postoperative period, the nurse will document the following daily and prn:
    - vital signs with systems review (neurologic, pulmonary, cardiac, circulatory, gastrointestinal, genitourinary, skin)
    - appearance of wound/dressings
    - color and amount of drainage/type of drains
    - intake and output
    - activity tolerance
    - comfort state, effectiveness of medication regimen, and nursing measures taken to enhance desired effects, or minimize side effects
    - nursing actions taken when early signs and symptoms of possible complications of abdominal surgery become evident (ie, unstable vital signs, excessive drainage/bleeding, nonfunctioning drains or tubes, nonrelieved pain, excessive vomiting, abdominal distention, signs and symptoms of infection, deterioration in mental status, evidence of altered venous flow in lower extremities, diminished breath sounds, and/or poor cough effort)
3. Before and after surgery, the nurse will document appropriate nursing diagnoses and individualized nursing approaches on the nursing care plan.
4. By discharge, the patient or caregiver will be able to
    - relate plan of care and its rationale
    - participate actively in the plan of care
    - identify resources (personal/community) available if assistance in that care is necessary

---

Adapted from Standards of Nursing Care for Patients Admitted for Abdominal Surgery, Paoli Memorial Hospital, Paoli, PA.

PRACTICE SESSION XII

Setting Priorities and Applying Standards

To complete this session, read pages 112–118. Example responses can be found on page 234.

1. What are the four main purposes of the plan of care?

Promotes communication between caregivers
Directs care and documentation
Creates a record that can later be used for eval, research, legal reasons
Provides documentation - insurance reimbursement

2. Name the three components of a plan of care and give an example of each.

Diagnoses/problems - self care deficit: dressing
Outcomes - will be able to dress self @ discharge
Interventions - have client practice buttoning shirt.

3. List five factors that may influence how you set priorities.

pt perception of priorities, understanding the whole pic of the problem, pts prognosis/health status, expected length of stay, presence of clinical guidelines

4. If you had someone with the following problems, which problem would you need to treat *immediately* and why?
   a. Diarrhea
   b. Severe dyspnea - severe breathing problems are top priority. unless hemoraging
   c. Risk for Fluid Volume Deficit

5. Give at least three types of standards that apply to your nursing practice.

State practice act
JCAHO
ANA standards

6. What is the relationship between setting priorities and identifying expected outcomes for discharge? Knowing expected outcomes makes it easy to prioritize to discharge in a timely fashion

Why Is Identifying Outcomes So Important?

Outcomes serve three main purposes:

1. **They're the measuring sticks of the plan of care.** You measure the success of the plan by determining whether the expected outcomes were met.

2. **They direct interventions.** You need to know *what* you're trying to accomplish before you can decide *how* to accomplish it.
3. **They're motivating factors.** Having a specific time frame for getting things done gets everyone in motion.

Determining Client-Centered Outcomes

Determining client-centered outcomes (what the *client* is expected to achieve) instead of nursing goals (what the *nurse* aims to achieve) is the key to outcome-based practice. If you focus on nursing goals (eg, I want to help this person feel better) instead of client outcomes (eg, what can I observe *in this person* to know if my treatments really are helping him feel better?), you basically monitor your *intentions*, not your *results*.

Client-centered outcomes focus on the desired result of treatment—that the *client* benefits from nursing care.

Remember the following rules.

RULE ▶

> The subject of a client-centered outcome must be either the client or a part of the client. For example, "*Chuck* will ambulate three times a day in the room."; "*The skin* will remain intact, free from signs of irritation."

RULE ▶

> The terms *goals, objectives,* and *outcomes* are often used interchangeably. However, *outcomes* are usually more *specific* and refer to *client* outcomes. To develop a very specific outcome, state the broad outcome, add "as evidenced by," and list the data that demonstrate outcome achievement. For example, "Will demonstrate knowledge of medication regimen *as evidenced by* ability to list drug names, actions, doses, and side effects.

Display 4–5 provides ANA standards related to identifying outcomes.

Study the following steps for deriving outcomes from nursing diagnoses.

Steps for Deriving Outcomes From Nursing Diagnoses

1. Look at the first clause of the nursing diagnosis or problem statement (the word or words before "related to").

EXAMPLE

> First Clause
>
> *Risk for Impaired Skin Integrity related to immobility*

DISPLAY 4–5 Standards for Outcomes (ANA, 1991)

Outcomes are:

- Derived from the diagnoses
- Documented as measurable goals
- Mutually formulated with the client and health care providers, when possible
- Realistic in relation to client's present and potential capabilities
- Attainable in relation to resources available to the client
- Written in such a way that they:

  Include a time estimate for attainment
  Provide direction for continuity of care

2. Now restate the first clause in a statement that describes improvement, control, or absence of the problem.

EXAMPLE

The person will demonstrate no signs of skin irritation or breakdown.

Table 4–1 on the next page gives two additional examples of outcomes derived from nursing diagnoses.

Think About It

At a simplistic level, developing outcomes requires you to simply reverse the problem. For example, if the person has such and such a problem, your desired outcome is that the person will not have that problem (or at least it will be greatly reduced).

Making Outcomes Clear and Specific

To be clear and specific, outcomes must have the following components:

Subject: Who is the person expected to achieve the outcome?
Verb: What actions must the person take to achieve the outcome?
Condition: Under what circumstances is the person to perform the actions?
Performance Criteria: How well is the person to perform the actions?
Target Time: By when is the person expected to be able to perform the actions?

EXAMPLE

Mr. Smith will walk with a cane at least to the end of the hall and back by Friday.

Subject: Mr. Smith
Verb: will walk
Condition: with a cane
Performance Criteria: at least to the end of the hall and back
Target Time: by Friday

TABLE 4–1 Example of Client Outcomes (Goals) Derived from Nursing Diagnoses

Nursing Diagnosis	Corresponding Client Outcome (Goal)
Ineffective Individual Coping	The client will demonstrate and relate effective coping as evidenced by self-report of coping better and ability to demonstrate good problem solving by March 1.
Constipation	The client will demonstrate normal bowel function as evidenced by having a normal stool every 1–2 days and by statements of feeling as though bowels are moving well by Jan 1.

Including the above five components creates a very specific outcome that can be used to identify interventions and monitor progress.

Choosing Measurable Verbs

When developing outcomes, choose verbs that are *measurable* (verbs that describe exactly what you expect to *see or hear* when the outcome has been achieved). For example, suppose you want someone to understand how to use sterile technique and you write an outcome that says, "Will understand how to use sterile technique." Experts would tell you that "will understand" is vague and not measurable. Ask yourself, "How can we really *know* if she understands?" The only way you can really know how well she understands is if she actually *verbalizes or demonstrates* sterile technique. Below are some examples of measurable verbs.

Measurable Verbs (Use these to be specific)

identify	hold	exercise
describe	demonstrate	communicate
perform	share	cough
relate	express	walk
state	will lose	stand
list	will gain	sit
verbalize	has an absence of	discuss

Nonmeasurable Verbs (Do not use)

know	think
understand	accept
appreciate	feel

Affective, Cognitive, and Psychomotor Outcomes

Outcomes are classified into three domains:

- *Affective Domain:* Outcomes associated with changes in attitudes, feelings, or values (eg, deciding old eating habits need to be changed).

- *Cognitive Domain:* Outcomes dealing with acquired knowledge or intellectual skills (eg, learning the signs and symptoms of diabetic shock).
- *Psychomotor Domain:* Outcomes dealing with developing motor skills (eg, mastering how to walk with crutches).

Table 4–2 shows examples of verbs that represent each domain.

Short-term Outcomes vs Long-term Outcomes

When someone requires long-term care, it may be appropriate to identify short-term outcomes (STO) and long-term outcomes (LTO). STOs are those that can be met relatively quickly, often in less than a week. LTOs are to be achieved over a longer period of time, often weeks or months.

Often you set several STOs to reach an LTO. For example, you may have an STO of "will walk the length of the hall with a walker by Friday," and an LTO of "will walk the length of the hall independently by the end of 2 weeks." LTOs may also include outcomes that are ongoing (ie, outcomes that are to be accomplished every day). For example, "Louise will dress herself every morning" or "Nat will maintain a fluid intake of 2000 ml a day."

The following guidelines summarize how to develop client-centered outcomes, whether they are long-term or short-term.

Guidelines: Determining Client-Centered Outcomes

- Be realistic, considering:
  - Physical health state, overall prognosis
  - Expected length of stay
  - Growth and development

EXAMPLE

Wrong: Tom will discuss the role of insulin in carbohydrate metabolism and give himself insulin.
Right: Tom will discuss the role of insulin in carbohydrate metabolism. Tom will give himself insulin.

TABLE 4–2 Examples of Verbs Representing the Three Domains

Cognitive	Affective	Psychomotor
Teach	Express	Demonstrate
Discuss	Share	Practice
Identify	Listen	Perform
Describe	Communicate	Walk
List	Relate	Administer
Explore		Give

  - ◦ Available human and material resources
  - ◦ Other planned therapies for the client
- Set goals mutually with the client and others involved in his health care (eg, significant others, other health care workers).
- When indicated, establish both short- and long-term outcomes.
- Be sure the outcomes describe something you can hear, see, or feel in the person that will demonstrate the desired control, resolution, or improvement of the person's problems.
- Be sure the outcomes you develop contain the five components listed on page 121.
- Use measurable, observable verbs (see page 122).
- Identify only one behavior per outcome. If you need to write two behaviors, write two outcomes.

Relationship of Outcomes and Accountability

Identifying outcomes helps you determine accountability. You look at the outcome and ask yourself, "Who's accountable for achieving this outcome?" If nursing is accountable for being the primary manager of the problem, then you're accountable for *initiating a comprehensive treatment plan.* If not, then you're accountable for *getting appropriate help.* The following diagram summarizes the decision-making process after you identify expected outcomes.

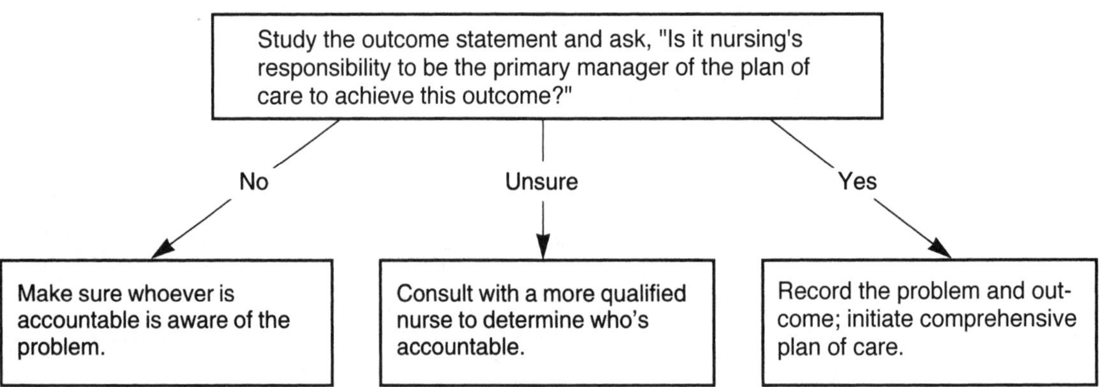

Accountability for Nursing Diagnoses and Collaborative Problems

As a nurse, you're solely accountable for achieving outcomes for nursing diagnoses, and you share accountability for achieving outcomes for collaborative problems with other members of the multidisciplinary team. For nursing diagnoses, you're accountable for initiating a plan *to detect and manage the problems.* For collaborative problems, your "share" of accountability includes initiating a plan *to monitor and detect signs and symptoms of potential complications.* For example, if you admit someone after surgery and you're concerned the person is at risk for hypotension, you're accountable for increasing the frequency of blood pressure measurements (eg, every hour) even if medical orders require only routine monitoring (eg, taking blood pressure every 4 hours). You're also accountable for implementing medical protocols and orders safely.

Clinical Outcomes for Collaborative/ Multidisciplinary Problems

Outcomes for collaborative problems are often covered on critical pathways, in an abbreviated form, as in the example below.

EXAMPLE

> Third Postoperative Day:
> Chest tube out (this demonstrates resolution of this problem)

If you're required to participate in writing clinical outcomes for multidisciplinary problems, keep in mind the following rule:

RULE ▶

> Clinical outcomes for multidisciplinary problems should reflect the desired status at discharge or at some other point in time. They should answer questions like, "What is the desired outcome 1 month after treatment began?" "What should be observed in the person?" "What is the desired health status (including absence or presence of disease), functional status, and quality of life?" See the following examples.

EXAMPLES OF CLINICAL OUTCOMES AT DIFFERENT POINTS IN TIME

> Four days after total knee replacement, Mr. Palmer (a police officer) will be discharged to a rehabilitation facility able to perform straight leg raises and range-of-motion exercises twice daily.
>
> Six months after total knee replacement, Mr. Palmer will return to work, able to perform usual job description (able to walk two to three flights of stairs, participate in a chase on foot, and so forth).

Case Management

Case management, which aims to minimize length of (or incidence of) hospital stays through early outcome identification, early detection of failure to achieve daily outcomes, and optimum use of resources, is an essential element of *Planning*. In today's health care arena, not only case managers are in charge of case management—*all nurses* in hospitals and communities must be attuned to people who demonstrate problems that might require additional resources to ensure efficient care. For example, suppose you assess someone who is to have a routine cholecystectomy, but is also paraplegic. This person is likely to have some additional care needs that an able-bodied person would not have. You should consider notifying a case manager *early* to ensure comprehensive planning aimed at preventing complications and achieving outcomes in a timely manner. Remember the following rule:

RULE ➧ Early in the planning phase, ask yourself, "Does this person have unusual health problems or disabilities that require close monitoring by a case manager?"

Discharge Outcomes and Discharge Planning

Identifying discharge outcomes early and starting discharge planning early are the hallmarks of efficiency. With today's decreased length of hospital stays, you must assess what will be needed when the person goes home as part of the *initial assessment*. Too often getting equipment and services needed for care upon discharge takes just as long as it takes the client to heal.

Usually, you record discharge outcomes in broad terms, describing the level of assistance the person is likely to need upon discharge (eg, "will be discharged home with care managed by wife and biweekly visits by home care nurse"). You may also record some very specific criteria about status of various problems (eg, "abdominal drains will be out," "wife will demonstrate care management of abdominal wound," and so forth).

Display 4–6 shows a discharge planning questionnaire that might be used to begin discharge planning.

Think About It

Discharge planning is at its best when it begins before admission and is kept simple. For example, going over a pathway for home care (Fig. 4–2) can teach people what to expect when they leave the hospital before they're in the midst of a stressful recovery.

DISPLAY 4–6 Discharge Planning Questionnaire

1. Is there a problem at home with any of the following?
   - Heat — Yes No Possibly
   - Hot/cold water — Yes No Possibly
   - Electricity — Yes No Possibly
   - Refrigeration — Yes No Possibly
   - Cooking — Yes No Possibly
   - Bathroom facilities — Yes No Possibly
   - Stairs
   - Wheelchair accessibility
2. Is necessary transportation available? — Yes No Possibly
3. Can the person be reached by phone? — Yes No Possibly

   If no, is there a neighbor who can be reached by phone? — Yes No Possibly
4. Will the patient/family require:

   Assistance with ADL — Yes No Possibly

   Assistance with medications — Yes No Possibly

   Assistance with treatments — Yes No Possibly

   Additional teaching — Yes No Possibly

   Ongoing nursing assessment — Yes No Possibly

   Community resources or referrals — Yes No Possibly

'AT HOME' PATH TO RECOVERY FROM CARDIAC SURGERY: THINGS TO DO EACH DAY				
Activity	*Health*	*Medications*	*Self-Care*	*Reasons to Call for More Information*
❑ Walk four times/day ❑ Do exercises as prescribed ❑ Rest ❑ Limit visitors the first week or so (three to four people for 30 minutes/day) ❑ Resume sexual activities when ready ❑ After two weeks, help with light housework	Do each of the following items around the same time each day: ❑ Check your incisions ❑ Take your temperature by mouth (call if over 100°F) 100° ❑ Check your pulse for one minute (normal: 60 to 120 beats/minute) ❑ Weigh yourself (call if you gain over 2 lb. in one day)	❑ Take your medications as prescribed ❑ Drink several glasses of water each day	❑ Keep your feet up while at rest ❑ Shower/bathe as instructed ❑ Practice reading food labels for fat intake, cholesterol, and sodium levels ❑ Eat healthy! Try new recipes ❑ Wear stockings if ordered	The nursing station phone number is (910) 716-6658. *Call your doctor if:* ❑ your heart rate (pulse) is less than 60 beats/minute or greater than 120 at rest, or ❑ you have severe chills, or ❑ unusual shortness of breath, or ❑ fever greater than 100°F (by mouth), or ❑ weight gain over 2 lb. in one day or 5 lb. in one week, or ❑ red or draining incisions, or ❑ chest pain, or ❑ if you have *any* questions or concerns

Source: Adapted from path developed by The North Carolina Baptist Hospitals, Winston-Salem, NC.

Figure **4–2.** Keeping pathways *simple* prevents people from being overwhelmed and promotes compliance (Wells, 1996).

PRACTICE SESSION XIII

Planning Outcome-Based Care

To complete this session, read pages 120–126. Example responses can be found on page 234.

Part I.

1. What are the three main purposes of outcomes? ① Measure sticks of the plan of care ② Direct interventions ③ Motivating factors for patients and care-givers. ① Evaluate progress

2. In nursing language, what three words are used interchangeably and usually mean the *desired result of* interventions?

Outcome, goal, objective

3. Of the three terms you listed above, which one is usually considered to be *most specific?* Outcome - most specific

4. a. If you identify an outcome and decide it's not within nursing's responsibility, what must you do? Report problem to person responsible in achieving outcome.

b. What must you do if it *is* within nursing's responsibility? Develop/initiate plan of care to treat problem

5. What are your responsibilities during planning in relation to case management? (Three sentences or less.) All nurses are responsible for detecting and reporting patients who may require case management.

Part II.

Measurable Verbs
Identify
Demonstrate
perform
Express

1. Why is it important to use measurable verbs when identifying outcomes? Give three examples of measurable verbs. Measurable verbs help everyone stay focused on observable data that will let you know how well the pt is progressing toward outcome achievement.

2. What are the five components of outcome statements? Subject, Verb, Condition, performance, and Target Time.

See pg 234

3. Choose the outcomes that are written correctly below. Identify what's wrong with the statements that are written incorrectly.

a. John will know the four basic food groups by 1/4.
Incorrect - the verb is not measurable.

subj verb Target time

b. Mrs. Eipert will demonstrate how to use her walker unassisted by Saturday.
Correct

c. Mr. McKillop will improve his appetite by 11/5.
nonspecific - how will we measure

d. Erica will list the equipment needed to change sterile dressings by 9/5.

Correct

e. Susan will walk independently in the hall the day after surgery.

Correct

f. Mrs. Baylis will understand the importance of maintaining a salt-free diet.

No time frame and verb is not measurable or observable

g. June will ambulate to the bathroom using her cane by 3/4.

Correct

h. Janet will lose 5 lb by 1/9.

Correct

i. Mr. Collins will feel less pain by Thursday.

rate pain

Verb isn't measurable

4. For each diagnosis or problem below, write an appropriate client outcome.

a. *Altered Oral Mucous Membrane related to poor oral hygiene.*

Will demonstrate healthy looking gums, without redness or irritation by Jan 15

b. *Risk for Impaired Skin Integrity related to constant diarrhea.*

Will not demonstrate signs/symptoms of impaired skin integrity in the rectal area and will be kept clear.

c. *English Impaired Verbal Communication related to inability to speak English.*

Will be able to communicate basic needs through use of flash cards and interpreter when required

Part III.

Identify whether each of the outcomes listed below is in the affective, cognitive, or psychomotor domain. Use "a" for affective, "c" for cognitive, and "p" for psychomotor. (Remember, there may be more than one domain for each outcome.)

a. Mrs. Resh will demonstrate how to sterilize her baby's formula.
b. Judy will relate her feelings concerning going home.
c. Mrs. Ballard will discuss the relationship between blood sugar levels and eating.
d. Connie will administer her own insulin according to the results of her morning blood sugar readings.

Part IV.

Once you've identified the domains of the outcomes in the above examples, write one or two activities that would help the client to achieve the outcome. (Note the example below.)

EXAMPLE

Sample outcome: Mrs. Jones will be able to dress herself without assistance by 7/4.
Domain: Psychomotor
Activities: Practice buttoning buttons and tying shoes on 7/1 and 7/2.
Practice putting on blouse, skirt, shoes, and socks on 7/3.
Demonstrate dressing herself on 7/4.

Determining Nursing Interventions

Nursing interventions are actions performed by the nurse to:

1. Monitor health status
2. Minimize risks
3. Resolve or control a problem.
4. Assist with activities of daily living (bathing and so forth).
5. Promote optimum health and independence.

Nursing interventions can be classified into two categories (ANA, 1995; McClosky & Bulechek, 1996):

Direct Care Interventions: Actions performed through interaction with clients. Some examples: helping someone out of bed, teaching someone about diabetes.

Indirect Care Interventions: Actions performed away from the client, but on behalf of a client or group of clients. These actions are aimed at managing the health care environment and promoting interdisciplinary collaboration. Some examples: monitoring lab study results, transferring a client from one room to another, contacting a social worker.

Classifying interventions into direct and indirect interventions helps account for nurses' time. If you focus only on what the nurse does directly with the client, you miss a lot of nursing time that's spent on other crucial nursing activities.

Assessment—Monitoring Health Status

Assessment may be planned specifically to detect or evaluate certain problems or to monitor responses to interventions. In fact, *Assessment* is a part of every intervention. Your plan should reflect awareness of the need to *assess before acting* to be sure the action is safe and appropriate, to assess *while acting* to monitor for adverse reactions, and to assess *after acting* to monitor the response. For example, if you get a man out of bed, you assess him before he gets out to be sure that he's still well enough to complete the activity, you monitor him for adverse reactions (eg, dizziness) as he's getting out of bed and is out of bed, and then you determine his *response* after he gets back into bed.

Think About It

Many nurses will tell you they spend more time assessing people, simply confirming that no problems exist, than they do actually treating problems. This is as it should be. When you carefully monitor health status, you're able to detect early signs and symptoms of potential problems, thereby reducing the amount of time spent treating the problems. Monitoring health status is time-consuming, but it takes only one disaster caused by that one time someone rushed through or skipped an assessment to make you realize it's worth every minute.

Teaching

Teaching may be planned specifically to enhance someone's knowledge about a specific problem (eg, teaching about diabetes) or as part of an intervention to explain why it's being done (eg, reinforcing the rationale for coughing and deep breathing as you're assisting the person to cough and breathe deeply). Teaching is an essential nursing intervention that should be employed at every opportunity. The following guidelines are suggested to help you plan teaching.

Guidelines: Planning Teaching

- Assess readiness to learn and previous knowledge before developing a teaching plan.
- Plan for a quiet, private environment conducive to learning.
- Identify active learning experiences (eg, use examples, simulations, games, and audiovisuals).
- Use simple terms: It's easy to overwhelm the average person.

- Determine learning outcomes mutually with the client so you both know what must be learned and mastered (eg, "How would you feel about learning how to give an injection by Thursday?").
- Encourage asking questions and verbalizing understanding of what is being taught (eg, "I want you to feel free to ask questions no matter how insignificant you think they are. It's not easy learning something new. It is very important that you understand this.").
- Plan to pace learning. Don't give too much information at one time; progress at the person's learning pace.
- Allow time to discuss progress (eg, to ask the person how he feels he's progressing) and to summarize what has been taught.
- Find ways to include significant others in the teaching session.

Counseling

Counseling people to help them make necessary changes in their lives or to help them make choices about their health care is another important nursing intervention. Counseling includes using teaching techniques to help people acquire the knowledge to make decisions about their health care. It also includes exploring motivations and offering support during periods of adjustment to new circumstances. By using teaching and therapeutic communication techniques, you can offer valuable psychological and intellectual support, thereby reducing the stress associated with making choices about health care management.

Consulting

Whenever problems require more than nurse-prescribed interventions, part of the plan must include consulting with, or referring to, the appropriate health care professional. For example, if someone has trouble swallowing pills, a nurse might consult with the pharmacist to determine if there's a better way of giving the medications (eg, a liquid form) or if someone isn't eating because she dislikes hospital food, contact the dietitian so different meals can be served.

Determining Nursing Orders

Determining nursing orders requires you to answer three key questions.

1. What can be done to prevent or minimize the *cause(s)* of this problem?
2. What can be done to minimize the *problem*?
3. How can I tailor interventions to meet this specific person's expected *outcome(s)*?

Figure 4–3 shows an example of how to apply the above questions to determine nursing orders for a specific nursing diagnosis and collaborative problem.

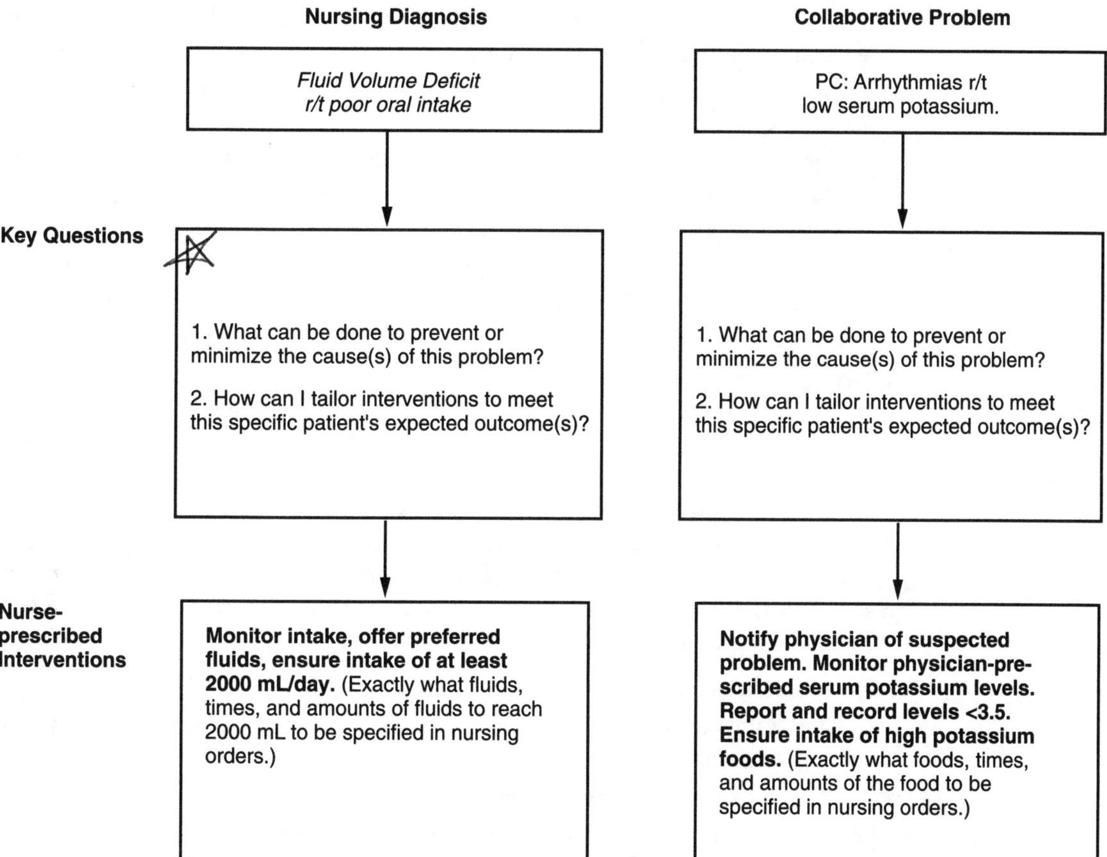

Figure **4–3.** Example of how to determine nurse-prescribed interventions for nursing diagnosis and a collaborative problem.

Guidelines: Determining Nursing Orders

- Determine a baseline of current signs and symptoms of the problem.
- Check for medical orders for nursing interventions related to the problem (eg, medications, diet, activity, diagnostic studies, and so forth).
- If you're using standard plans (eg, critical path, preprinted plan, protocol):
  - Use them with a critical mind. Compare the person's specific situation with the standard plan. Decide what applies, what doesn't, and what's missing.
  - Modify (add, delete, change) interventions as indicated, depending on your current assessment findings and what's likely to work for this specific person.
- Identify monitoring regimens for potential complications: What will you monitor? How often will you monitor it? How often will you record assessment data?

- Identify interventions that prevent or minimize the underlying cause(s) of the problem and help achieve the expected outcome.
- If you can't do anything about the *cause,* decide if there's anything that can be done about the *problem.*
- Be sure the interventions are congruent with other therapies (eg, allow for rest after physical therapy).
- Consider the person's preferences; individualize as much as possible.
- Determine the scientific rationale for planned actions.
- Create opportunities for teaching (eg, explain rationale for all actions).
- Consult with other professionals when indicated (physician, ARNP, physical therapist).
- Before prescribing any actions:
  - Weigh the risks and benefits of performing the actions (Display 4–7).
  - Decide whether you're willing to be accountable for the responses to the interventions you prescribe.
- Make your orders specific: Keep in mind "see, do, teach, record" (ie, what to assess (see), what to do, what to teach, and what to record). For example, suppose you're caring for someone who's had abdominal surgery, and you identify *Risk for Ineffective Airway Clearance related to history of smoking and incision pain.* Your orders might look like this:

  1. Auscultate lungs every 4 hours.
  2. Assist the person to perform coughing and breathing exercises with pillow and hand over incision every 4 hours.
  3. Reinforce the importance of coughing and deep breathing.
  4. Record lung sounds and sputum production once a shift and prn.

What You Should Include in Your Nursing Orders

Date: The date the order was written
Verb: Action to be performed.
Subject: Who is to do it.
Descriptive Phrase: How, when, where, how often, how long, or how much?
Signature: Be consistent in how you sign.

Example: (today's date) Assist Chelsey to stand by the side of the bed for 10 minutes twice a day wearing her back brace. R. Alfaro-LeFevre RN

Carrying Out Medical Orders Safely and Effectively

When physicians or ARNPs prescribe medical interventions, they rely on your nursing judgment and skill in carrying them out. You're responsible for acting independently to ensure that orders are carried out safely and effectively. Before carrying out medical orders, be clear about the following:

1. What action(s) is to be performed.
2. Why the action(s) is to be performed.
3. How it's to be performed.
4. When and how often it's to be performed.
5. How much and, in the case of medications, how long and by what route will the intervention be performed.

If you're unclear about any of the above, make sure you clarify the orders.

Documenting the Plan of Care

Forms for, and methods of, documenting care plans are tailor-made to meet the needs of the nurses and clients in each unique setting. As you move from one facility to another, you'll need to familiarize yourself with their particular policies for recording a plan of care. However, keep in mind that to meet current standards of care, somewhere on the medical record, evidence of the following must be found:

- The most important client problems (those that will be resolved or improved by discharge).
- Interventions planned to meet the client's needs, including teaching and discharge planning needs.
- Expected outcomes of care.

DISPLAY 4-7 Weighing Risks Against Benefits

Weigh the risks of *causing harm* against the probability of *reducing the problem* by prescribing an intervention as a habit of safe practice. Once you've identified an intervention, ask the following questions:

1. If I prescribe this intervention, how likely are we to see the desired response?
2. What is the worst thing that can happen if this intervention is performed, and how likely is it to happen?
3. What measures can be taken to minimize the chances of causing harm?
4. What would happen to this problem if *no* intervention(s) were prescribed?

By answering the above questions and considering the possible responses, you can *weigh the risks* (of prescribing the interventions and having an adverse reaction, or allowing the problem to go untreated) *against the benefits* (the likelihood of achieving the desired response) if the intervention is performed. Answering the above four questions will help you choose the safest intervention(s) and be prepared if an adverse reaction happens.

Computerized Care Planning and Standard Plans

More facilities are using computerized care planning and other standard plans to make the process more efficient. Because these types of care planning are constantly changing, you must be committed to learning new methods and understanding the rationale behind them. Also remember that these plans aren't intended to *think* for you. They're intended to be used *as guides* to care. As the nurse, you're responsible for:

- Detecting changes in client status that may contraindicate following the plan.
- Using good judgment about which parts of the plans apply and which do not.
- Recognizing when problems aren't covered by the plan, (and finding another way to address them).

Computerized and standard plans may be based on medical diagnoses or nursing diagnoses. If the person has more than one major problem, you may need to use more than one applicable plan, or choose the most relevant plan and modify it. The important thing to remember is that these types of plans are developed for specific *problems,* not people, and you *must* be sure you carefully adapt any standard plan to the person's *specific situation.*

Remember the following rule:

RULE ➧ As a nurse, you're responsible for making sure that any problem or diagnosis that's likely to impede progress toward outcome achievement is addressed somewhere on the plan of care. This may require adapting a standard plan, adding a standard plan, or developing an additional plan of your own.

Multidisciplinary Plans

Multidisciplinary plans, in which all disciplines (medicine, dietary, and so forth) work from the same plan, are the norm in many facilities. Multidisciplinary approaches often bring "the best of all worlds" together. However, keep in mind that, as the nurse, you're with the person 8 hours a day. You're in the best position to be realistic about how the plan will come together *as a whole,* on a day-by-day, hour-by-hour basis. It's your job to stay focused on *human responses,* how the person is likely to *respond as a whole* to the plan of care, and to act as a client advocate.

Pages 137 through 146 provide examples of various care plans. Student plans are sometimes more theoretical and comprehensive because they're used to assess the student's knowledge of nursing theory and all aspects of nursing process.

(text continued on page 146)

NURSING CARE PLAN

Date	Nursing Diagnosis	Expected Outcomes	Target Date	Resol Date
	Ineffective Breathing Pattern related to neuro-muscular impairment	(1) Achieve optimal lung expansion with adequate ventilation.	LTO	
	as evidenced by C-6 spinal cord injury, poor chest expansion	X Identify causative factors and relate adaptive ways of coping with them.	Strength: Knows this well.	
		(3) Remain free of signs and symptoms of hypoxia.	LTO	
	Commmon Etiologies Neuromuscular Impairment Pain Musculoskeletal Impairment Inflammatory Process Anxiety Decreased Lung Expansion Decreased Energy or Fatigue Infection Tracheo-Bronchial Obstruction Structural Damage	(4) Relate relief of symptoms and comfort in breathing. (5) Demonstrates effective breathing techniques and use of assistive devices.	LTO LTO	

Figure **4–4.** Sample page from a nursing care plan that uses a separate page for each nursing diagnosis. Adapted with permission of Bryn Mawr Hospital, Bryn Mawr, Pa.

Nursing Interventions	Date IMP/DC	Nursing Orders	Date IMP/DC
1. Assess causative or contributing factors.	5/10	- Auscultate lungs q 4° + prn + chart q 8°.	5/10 RA
2. Reduce or eliminate causative or contributing factors, if possible.	5/10	- Monitor use of incentive spirometer (he tries to skip when he's tired).	5/10 RA
3. Assist patient in use of respiratory devices and techniques.	5/10		
4. Provide for adequate rest periods between treatments.	5/10	- Reinforce need for practicing quad cough.	5/10 RA
5. Promote comfort.	5/10	- Encourage family to help him to ↑ mobility and to turn from side to side.	5/10 RA
6. Provide emotional support.	5/10		
7. Maintain adequate ventilation.	5/10		
8. Assess for signs and symptoms of hypoxia.	5/10	- Document vital capacity q 8 hours on flow sheet.	5/10 RA
9. Initiate health teaching and referrals as indicated.	5/10	- Record daily teaching on discharge planning sheet.	5/10 RA

Figure 4–4. *(Continued)*

Community Nursing Service & Hospice

CLIENT'S NAME ______________ PLACE LABEL HERE
FID # ______________

INTERDISCIPLINARY CARE PLAN

(Page 1 of 4)

Physician ______________ Address ______________

1. Diagnosis(es): Principal ______________
   Secondary

2. Mental Status (check one)
   ☐ Alert ☐ Lethargic ☐ Other
   ☐ Semicomatose ☐ Comatose

3. Prognosis and Rehabilitation Potential

4. Diet

5. Homebound Status/Functional Limitations

6. Safety Precautions

7. Supplies/Equipment

8. Medications

Name	Dosage	Frequency

9. Frequency of Visits/Duration of Service
   a. Skilled Nursing ______________
   b. Home Health Aide ______________
   c. MD ______________
   d. Social Service ______________
   e. Volunteer ______________
   f. Clergy ______________
   g. Other ______________

PROBLEM: Incomplete adjustment by client/S.O.(s) to effects of the terminal illness on the family unit.	Date Recorded	Date Resolved	Person(s) Responsible

GOAL: Enhance quality of life for client/S.O.(s) during the dying process.

PLAN:

☐ 1. Present Hospice philosophy and services.
☐ 2. Assess client/S.O.(s) wishes and expectations regarding care.
☐ 3. Assess client, significant other, or caregiver resources available for care and encourage or supplement their use.
☐ 4. Assess psychosocial reaction of client/S.O.(s) to client's prognosis.
☐ 5. Encourage client/S.O.(s) to get legal and personal affairs in order.
☐ 6. Discuss and support intervention for alleviating fears, stress, etc., and encourage verbalization of feelings as family and/or client expresses the need.
☐ 7. Discuss signs and symptoms of impending death and what to do to promote comfort in dying.
☐ 8. ______________

Cert Period from ______________ to ______________

12. Review Frequency:

13. Dates Plan Reviewed
    1) ______ 2) ______ 3) ______ 4) ______ 5) ______
    6) ______ 7) ______ 8) ______ 9) ______ 10) ______

Case Manager's Signature	Hospice Medical Director's Signature	Attending Physician's Signature
Date Signed:	Date Signed:	Date Signed:

CNS377 2/93

Figure **4–5.** Care Plan. (Courtesy of Community Nursing Service, Salt Lake City, Utah.)

Community Nursing Service & Hospice

CLIENT'S NAME ______________
FID # ______________

PLACE LABEL HERE

INTERDISCIPLINARY CARE PLAN
(Page 2 of 4)

PROBLEM: Alteration in comfort. ☐ Skin ☐ HEENT ☐ Cardiopulmonary ☐ GI ☐ GU ☐ MS ☐ CNS	Date Recorded	Date Resolved	Person(s) Responsible

GOALS:
1. Client/S.O. expresses verbally or nonverbally increased level of comfort.
2. Client/S.O. will be able to apply measures to control symptom(s) effectively and safely.

PLAN:
- ☐ 1. Assess pain and other symptoms, including site, duration, characteristics and relief measures.
- ☐ 2. Teach caregiver symptom control and relief measures.
- ☐ 3. Teach new pain and symptom control medication regimen and effects of medications.
- ☐ 4. Diet counseling for patients with anorexia.
- ☐ 5. Assess bowel regimen and implement as needed.
- ☐ 6. Check for and remove impaction as needed.
- ☐ 7. Fleets or tap water enema as needed.
- ☐ 8. Rectal tube for increased flatulence.
- ☐ 9. Assess mental status and sleep disturbance changes.
- ☐ 10. Oxygen on at ______ liters per ______. Teach safety.
- ☐ 11. ______________________________

PROBLEM: Self-care deficit.	Date Recorded	Date Resolved	Person(s) Responsible

GOALS:
1. Caregiver able to care for client at home.
2. ADL's and personal hygiene met through agency staff assistance.

PLAN:
- ☐ 1. Teach client/S.O. safety measures.
- ☐ 2. Teach S.O. care of weak, terminally ill client.
- ☐ 3. Teach care of the bedridden client.
- ☐ 4. Teach client/S.O. regarding techniques for energy conservation.
- ☐ 5. Teach catheter care.
- ☐ 6. HHA to assist with ADL's and personal hygiene. See care plan.
- ☐ 7. Teach feeding tube care to S.O.
- ☐ 8. Teach S.O.: ☐ p.o. ☐ s.l. ☐ topical ☐ rectal ☐ s.q. ☐ i.m. ☐ i.v. technique for medication administration.
- ☐ 9. ______________________________

CNS377 2/93

Figure **4–5.** *(Continued)*

Community Nursing Service & Hospice

CLIENT'S NAME ____________ PLACE LABEL HERE
FID # ____________

INTERDISCIPLINARY CARE PLAN
(Page 3 of 4)

PROBLEM: Technical Deficit	Date Recorded	Date Resolved	Person(s) Responsible

GOALS: Professional disease management in the home.
PLAN:
☐ 1. Assess disease process progression and address with all involved members of the Interdisciplinary Team.
☐ 2. Assess for electrolyte imbalance.
☐ 3. Assess amount and frequency of urinary output.
☐ 4. Assess skin integrity.
☐ 5. Assess weight.
☐ 6. Assess for edema.
☐ 7. Measure abdominal girth.
☐ 8. Assess cardiovascular, pulmonary and respiratory status.
☐ 9. Assess nutrition and hydration status.
☐ 10. Measure vital signs.
☐ 11. Assess S.O.(s) knowledge and skill regarding technical procedures and care giving.
☐ 12. Administer: ☐ p.o. ☐ s.l. ☐ topical ☐ rectal ☐ s.q. ☐ i.m. ☐ i.v. ☐ injection ☐ infusion for symptom control.
☐ 13. ☐ Condom or ☐ indwelling catheter, size ______, insertion and maintenance. Change every ______ or when leaking or plugged.
☐ 14. Decubitus care (describe): ____________
☐ 15. Dressing change (describe): ____________
☐ 16. Obtain venipuncture for ____________
☐ 17. Record and report significantly abnormal findings to physician.
☐ 18. Do not attempt resuscitation.
☐ 19. ____________

BEREAVEMENT

PROBLEM: Potential/actual failure of survivors to complete bereavement process.	Date Recorded	Date Resolved	Person(s) Responsible

GOALS: To provide appropriate intervention for surviving family members, S.O. and IDT members to facilitate progression of the bereavement process within one year of the client's death.
PLAN:
☐ 1. Present hospice bereavement philosophy and services to S.O.
☐ 2. Assess S.O.'s response and reactions, coping strategies, support systems available, risk of pathological grief reactions, and desire of survivors for bereavement follow-up within the first week of service.
☐ 3. Invite S.O. to bereavement support group within first month following the client's death.
☐ 4. Contact S.O. at 3, 6, 9, and 12 months following the client's death.
☐ 5. Refer S.O. demonstrating pathological grief reactions to appropriate community resources.
☐ 6. Reassess S.O.'s adjustment at 12 months following the client's death and discharge from Hospice program if appropriate.

CNS377 2/93

Figure **4–5.** *(Continued)*

Community Nursing Service & Hospice

CLIENT'S NAME ______________
FID # ______________
PLACE LABEL HERE

INTERDISCIPLINARY CARE PLAN
(Page 4 of 4)

IN-PATIENT PAIN AND SYMPTOM MANAGEMENT AND RESPITE

PROBLEM:	Date Recorded	Date Resolved	Person(s) Responsible
☐ A. Symptoms. Specify: ______________, ______________, ______________. ☐ B. Client care in home.			

GOALS:
1. To institute program for ______________, ______________, ______________, management to be continued at home.
2. To allow caregiver respite time to enhance coping ability.
3. To assure continuity of care.

PLAN:
☐ 1. Assess need through interdisciplinary team discussion.
☐ 2. Contact and coordinate care with contracted in-patient facility to assure continuity of care.
☐ 3. Establish plan of care with in-patient staff for in-patient stay.
☐ 4. Contact in-patient staff and client/S.O. regarding progression towards care plan goals daily. Visit at least every other day.
* ☐ 5. Facilitate safe return to the home setting.

*Transportation is the family's responsibility.

Case Manager's Signature	Hospice Medical Director's Signature	Attending Physician's Signature
Date Signed:	Date Signed:	Date Signed:

CNS377 2/93

Figure **4–5.** *(Continued)*

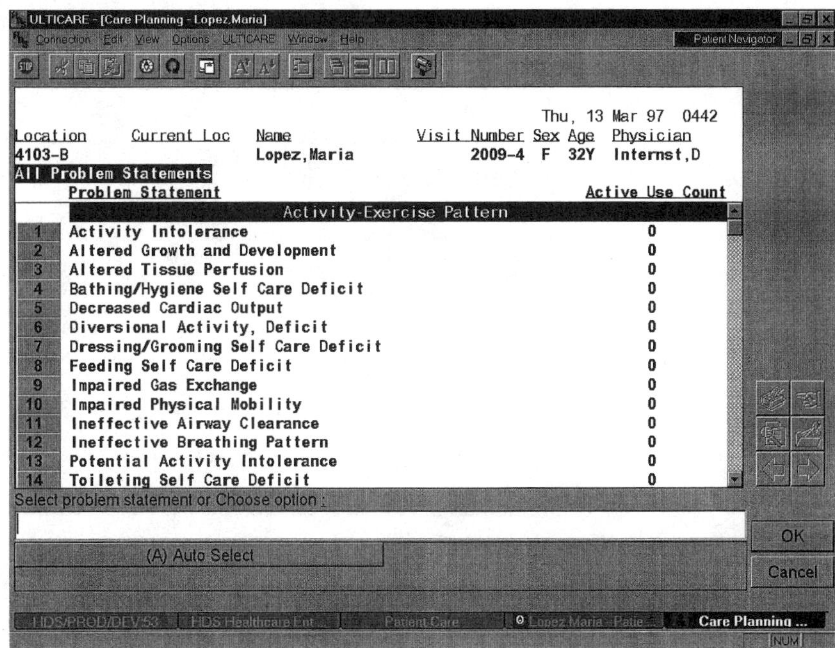

Figure 4–6. Suggested possible NANDA nursing diagnoses based on documentation assessments. (Courtesy of Health Data Sciences Corporation, San Bernardino, Calif.)

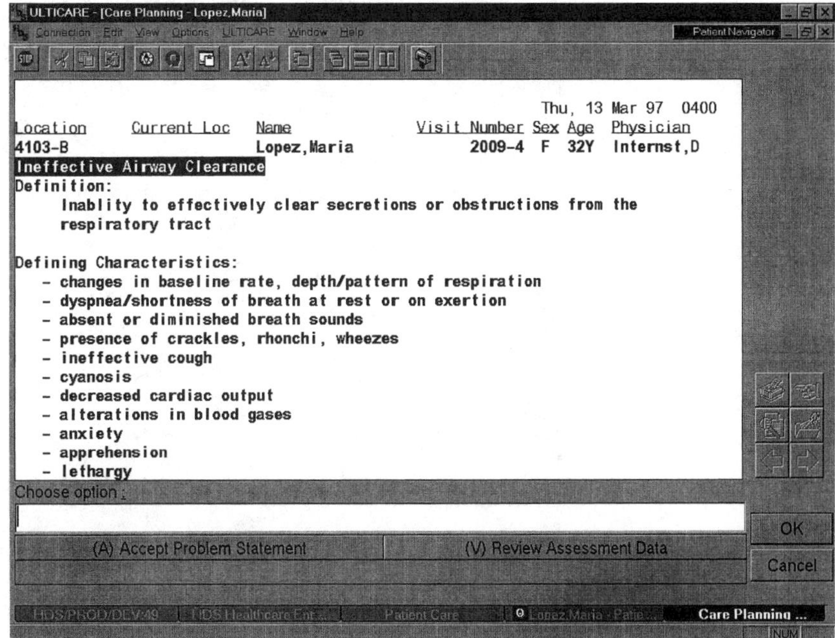

Figure 4–7. Once a NANDA diagnosis is selected, the definition and defining characteristics are displayed. (Courtesy of Health Data Sciences Corporation, San Bernardino, Calif.)

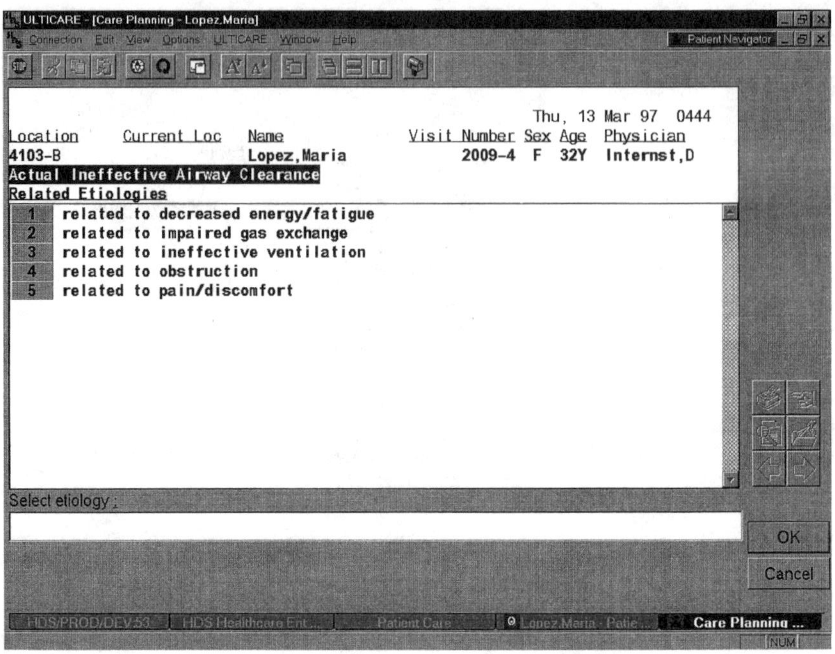

Figure **4–8.** After a NANDA diagnosis is selected, the system prompts for a related factor. (Courtesy of Health Data Sciences Corporation, San Bernardino, Calif.)

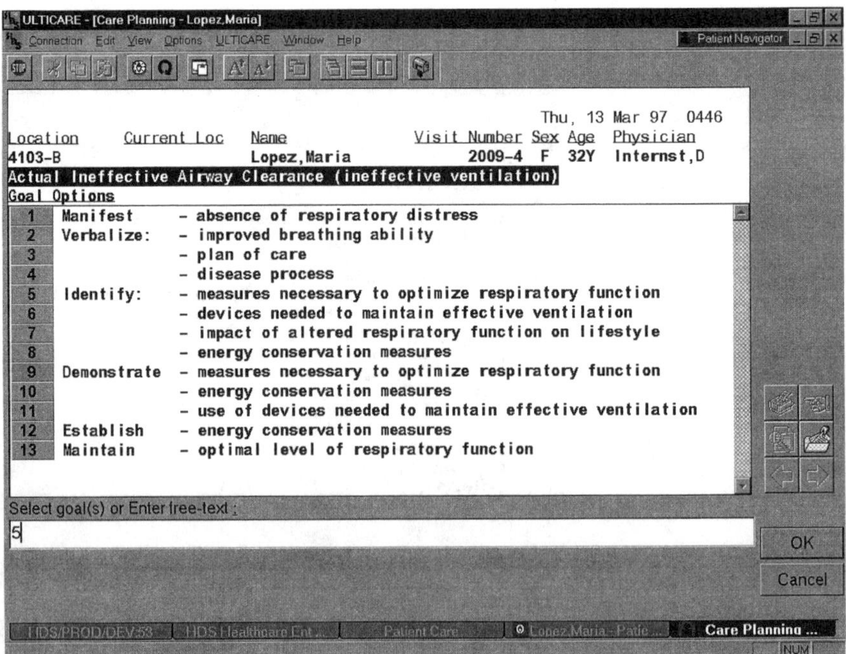

Figure **4–9.** Once a NANDA diagnosis and related factor are selected, the system prompts for outcomes. (Courtesy of Health Data Sciences Corporation, San Bernardino, Calif.)

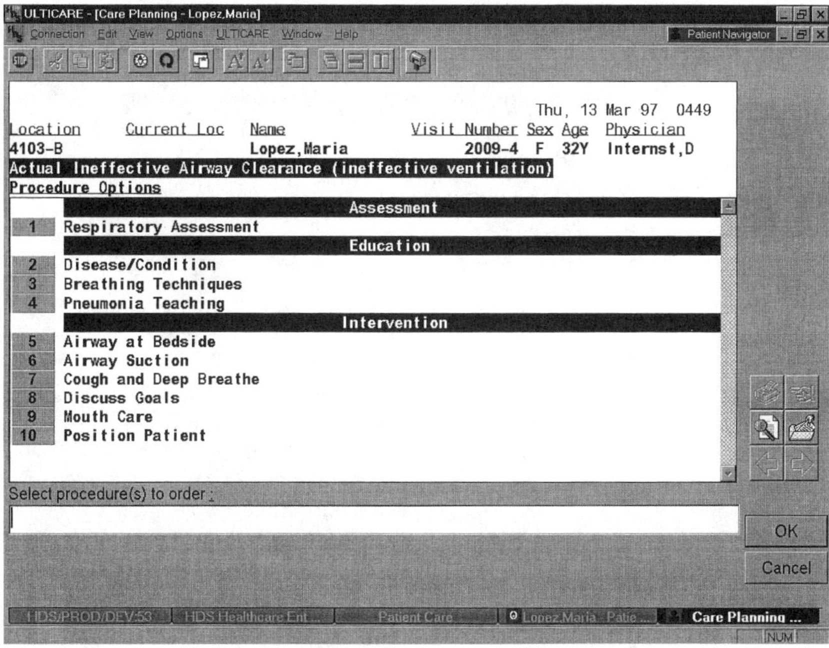

Figure **4–10.** Next, nursing interventions are displayed. (Courtesy of Health Data Sciences Corporation, San Bernardino, Calif.)

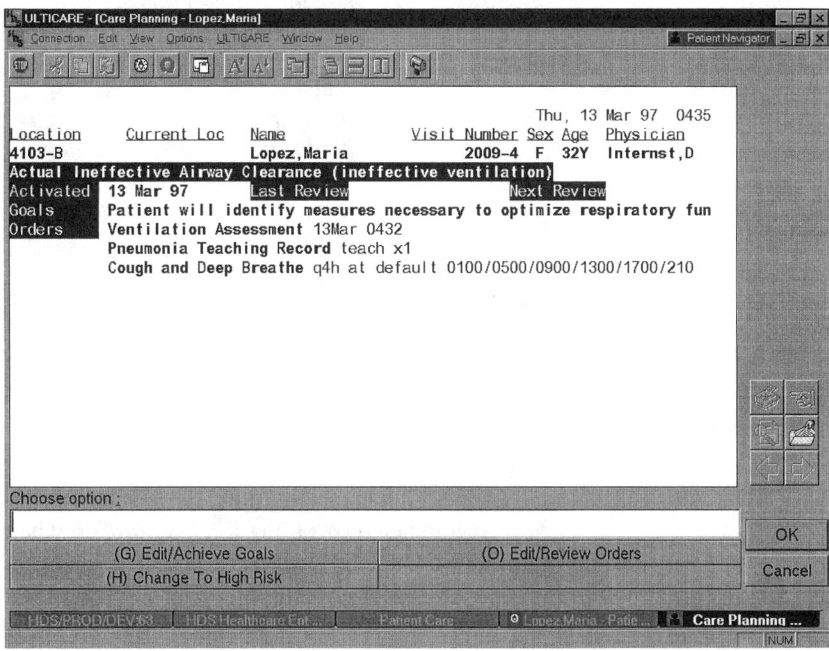

Figure **4–11.** A completed care plan is shown. (Courtesy of Health Data Sciences Corporation, San Bernardino, Calif.)

DISPLAY 4-8 Multidisciplinary Record & SOAP Charting

Description: Sample of a multidisciplinary record, where all disciplines chart on the same record, creating an interdisciplinary problem list (see I below) and sample of SOAP charting (see II below).

I. Sample problem list

Date of Diagnosis	Problem	Date Resolved
1/5	1. *Cerebrovascular accident* (identified by physician)	
	2. *Risk for Impaired Skin Integrity related to immobility* (identified by nursing)	
	3. Unsteady gait (identified by physical therapist)	
1/7	4. *Body Image Disturbance* (identified by nursing)	
1/8	5. *Urinary tract infection* (identified by physician)	1/13

II. Sample SOAP charting.*

S: Subjective Data	"I can't feel anything on the right side."
O: Objective Data	Absent reflexes on right side. Slouched in bed, leaning toward right. Has reddened area about 5 cm on right hip.
A: Analysis	*Risk for Impaired Skin Integrity related to right-sided loss of sensation and immobility.*
P: Plan	Prevent skin breakdown. Monitor back and hips for signs of decreased circulation from pressure point every 2 hours. Reposition side, back, side every 2 hours. Place air mattress and sheepskin on bed.

*After initial planning, some facilities add I (implementation) and E (evaluation), making the acronym SOAPIE.

Critical Thinking: Evaluating Early

Once you've completed recording the plan of care, take some time to evaluate what you've produced. Comprehensive care planning is a complicated process. Early evaluation of what you've produced promotes critical thinking by helping you detect oversights and errors early. For example, use checklist in Display 4–9 to decide how your plan "measures up."

DISPLAY 4–9 Checklist to Evaluate the Initial Plan of Care

- Was the plan developed with the client (and, if appropriate, significant others and other involved health care providers)?
- Have you listed the problems requiring individualized, not routine nursing interventions?
- If you've identified problems that aren't on the plan of care, have you ensured that they are addressed somewhere in the patient's record (eg, chest tube management might be addressed by physician's orders)?
- Are the outcomes:

  Derived from the diagnoses or problems?
  Measurable?
  Mutually formulated?
  Realistic and attainable?
  Written according to the rules (client-centered, measurable verbs, clear about who, what, when, how, and where, directive of interventions, inclusive of a time-frame for goal achievement)?
- Do the nursing orders:

  Include interventions that focus on treating the *underlying cause* of the problem (or, if that's not possible, treating the *problem*)?
  Clearly direct interventions (addressing who, what, when, how, and how much, as appropriate)?
  Incorporate use of resources and strengths?
  Indicate the signature of whoever prescribed the orders?
- Does the plan:

  Reflect current nursing practice?
  Provide for continuity?

PRACTICE SESSION XIV

Determining and Recording Nursing Orders

To complete this session, read pages 130–147. Example responses can be found on page 235.

Part I.

1. What's the point of classifying interventions into direct and indirect interventions? (3 sentences or less.) It allows you to examine nursing activities and time spent in direct contact c̄ patients and activities and time spent performing activities on patients behalf, but away from the patient

2. How do the words "see, do, teach, record" help you remember what you need to consider when determining interventions?

See = what must be assessed or observed related to the intervention. Do = what must be done
Teach = what must be taught or reinforced
Record = what must be recorded related to intervention

3. After you identify a problem, what 2 questions do you need to ask to determine interventions?

- what can be done about the cause of this problem
- what can be done to help this specific person achieve this specific outcome

4. Explain how to weigh risks and benefits. (5 sentences or less.)

intervention → desired outcome
worst thing

Part II.

For each nursing diagnosis and outcome listed below, list some possible nursing interventions that would help the client to reach the goal.

1. **Nursing Diagnosis:** *Risk for Impaired Skin Integrity related to prescribed bed rest and loss of sensation in lower extremities.*
   Outcome: Will maintain healthy-looking skin while on bed rest as evidenced by absence of redness or breakdown.
   List appropriate nursing interventions:

   Turn q2
   air mattress
   clean/dry/unwrinkled sheets

2. **Nursing Diagnosis:** *Risk for Ineffective Airway Clearance related to thoracic, incision pain.*
   Outcome: Will demonstrate effective airway clearance as evidenced by the ability to clear lungs with coughing.
   List appropriate nursing interventions.

   Teach importance of pain med.
   early walking, coughing, deep breathing

3. **Nursing Diagnosis:** *Constipation related to insufficient exercise and inadequate fluid and roughage intake as evidenced by no BM in 4 days.*
   Outcome: Will have daily soft bowel movements as evidenced by patient report.
   List appropriate nursing interventions.

   Monitor dly bowel movements
   increase fld intake, diet, exercise

Part III.

When working with collaborative problems, a major independent responsibility of the nurse is to monitor for potential complications. For each of the collaborative problems below, identify potential complications and determine how, and how often you plan to monitor for the problems. (You may need to use an additional resource, such as a medical-surgical textbook for this section.)

1. Intravenous infusion at 25 mL/h
Potential complications:

Plan for monitoring to detect potential complications:

2. Insulin-dependent diabetes.
Potential complications:

Plan for monitoring to detect potential complications:

3. Foley catheter.
Potential complications:
Infection, Bleeding
Blocking of catheter

Plan for monitoring to detect potential complications: I&O q8
cath care
monitor temp q4-8h
monitor urine color, amt, odor

Try This on Your Own

Try weighing risks and benefits and making decisions about interventions. Consider the following interventions and decide whether you'd prescribe them and whether there was anything you could do to minimize the risks involved.

1. Your neighbor calls at 10 PM and tells you her 9-year-old has chickenpox and is generally irritable and uncomfortable. She asks you if you think it would be okay to give her Children's Tylenol. What would you tell her? What would you have told her if it were *aspirin*? Be sure to look these drugs up before answering.
2. Mr. Ogden is weak from being on bed rest. He reports being depressed because he's become so dependent on others. He's now allowed to go to the bathroom on his own, and requests that he be allowed to do his daily hygiene unsupervised in the bathroom. You are concerned that he might tire in the bathroom. Would you prescribe for him to be allowed to do his morning care alone in the bathroom? If, so what would you do to minimize the risks?
3. Your patient has a left chest tube and doesn't want to lie tilted to his left side because it's painful. Even though his right lung is compromised from previous disease process, he insists on being turned only to the right side. Would you allow him to turn only to his right side? If so, what would you do to minimize the risks?

Summary

Methods of developing and recording the plan of care continue to change as health care providers seek to be more efficient. Multidisciplinary approaches bring "the best of all worlds" to care planning. The plan benefits from the expert input of different professionals. As we continue to change, remember that, no matter what care planning method you use, to meet today's standards, the plan of care must be able to answer all the following questions:

What are the problems that must be prevented, resolved, or improved by the time of discharge?

What are the expected outcomes?

What are the interventions required to prevent, resolve, or control the status of the problems?

When indicated, the plan must also give special attention to teaching needs and discharge planning.

Evaluate your knowledge of this chapter. Check to see if you can achieve the objectives on page 110.

Bibliography: See pages 189–191.

CHAPTER 5

Implementation

OBJECTIVES

Once you complete this chapter, you should be able to:

- Identify ways you can be more prepared for getting change-of-shift report the next time you're in the clinical setting.
- Explain the importance of assessing and reassessing when implementing a plan of care.
- Discuss how you'll set daily priorities the next time you're in the clinical setting.
- Explain how to decide whether to delegate an action to an unlicensed helper.
- Address your accountability in relation to delegating actions.
- Describe how to reduce the likelihood of harm from an intervention.
- Address your role in relation to case management and variances in care.
- Describe the characteristics of effective charting systems.
- Chart effectively following guidelines from the facility you'll go to for your next clinical assignment.
- Discuss how you'll give a factual, organized change-of-shift report the next time you're in the clinical setting.

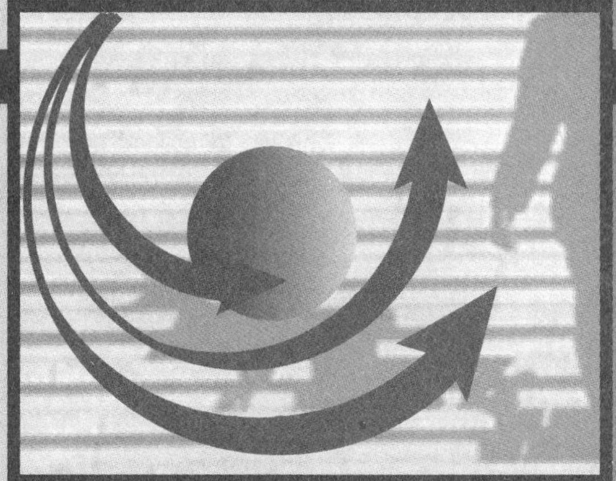

Standard I. *Assessment.* The nurse collects client health data.

Standard V. *Implementation.* The nurse implements interventions identified in the plan of care.

Standard VI. *Evaluation.* The nurse evaluates the client's progress toward attainment of outcomes.*

Practice Sessions

- **Practice Session XV:** Delegating, Case Management, Critical Paths, and Care Variances.
- **Practice Session XVI:** Principles of Effective Charting

What's in this chapter?

Whereas the last chapter addressed how to develop an initial comprehensive plan of care, this chapter focuses on the daily activities of *putting the plan into action.* It suggests steps for setting priorities and answers the question "When and how is it appropriate to delegate care to others?". It stresses the need to monitor responses to interventions by assessing and reassessing as you carry out the plan, and provides guidelines for charting effectively (creating a record that clearly shows what happened, when it happened, where it happened, and how it happened).

---

*Excerpted from ANA Standards of Clinical Nursing Practice (1991).

Putting the Plan Into Action

You've developed the plan. Now you're ready for *Implementation,* or *putting the plan into action. Implementation* includes:

- Preparing for report and getting report
- Setting daily priorities
- Assessing and reassessing
- Performing interventions and making necessary changes
- Charting
- Giving report

Let's go through each of these activities step by step.

Preparing for Report and Getting Report

In the clinical setting, you're often not involved in the initial planning. Rather, you begin taking care of people after *Planning* has been completed and *Implementation* has already begun—you get report from someone who's been implementing the plan in your absence. Being prepared and staying focused can be the key to getting a factual, relevant report that helps you get organized and set priorities early in the day.

Preparing for Report

Preparing for report—learning about patient problems and common treatments, reading charts, and getting to the unit early—can be the key to efficiency in today's rapidly changing workplace. All too often there's little time for reading charts and looking up management of common problems during the course of the day. When you have time to prepare yourself for the day, you feel more confident, *are* more competent, and can begin giving care in a timely fashion.

Getting Report

Getting a factual, relevant report can be quite a challenge for several reasons: there are often interruptions and distractions as one shift ends and the other begins; there's so much information that it's hard to write quickly enough; nurses giving report are often fatigued, or they may know the patients so well that they forget to tell you unique aspects of care that you may need to know.

Coming to report with a prepared worksheet helps you stay focused and get the necessary facts. For example, look at Figure 5–1, which shows the worksheet I developed for myself when I was working part-time in an intensive care unit (ICU). Note how the preprinted worksheet directs the questions you may need to ask in an ICU and saves time by providing information you'd otherwise have to write out in long hand.

Name Wm. French	Room: 145
Age 62	Med Dx: Angina
Dr. O'Hara	Nsg Dx: Activity Intolerance
Mental Status: ok	Diet: Reg. No Caf
Airway: ok	IV: Hep lock @ hand
Lungs: clear	Pain? None since yesterday
Oxygen: at 2 l per cannula	Relevant History Hypertension
Heart rhythm: reg - no PVC's	
GI: ok	
GU: ok	Special Concerns - For stress test tomorrow - Wants to see priest for communion
Skin: ok	
Activity Restrictions: OOB to chair only	
EKG: ok Na ok Cl ok K 3.5 CO_2 ok	
VITAL SIGNS: 98⁴-72-22 140/90	BLD SUGAR: ok
BLOOD GASES: ok	O_2 SATURATION: ok

Figure **5–1.** Sample report worksheet. Use back of sheet for additional notes.

Preprinted worksheets serve several purposes:

- You can get more information down quickly.
- You organize the information as you fill in the blanks (this is especially helpful when information is reported *to you* in a disorganized way).

- You can readily identify when information is omitted (areas that are blank jog your memory about pertinent questions to ask).
- You can use the worksheet for notes during the day, and later, when you give report, you can be more organized and comprehensive by systematically covering all the categories on the sheet.

If you don't have a preprinted worksheet, develop one yourself, and use it consistently. You'll be surprised how it will help you be more organized.

Setting Daily Priorities

Setting priorities during *Implementation* requires applying the same principles of priority setting you learned in *Planning* (page 113). However, the steps for setting priorities on a daily basis are a little different because *Implementation* focuses more on *doing* than planning.

Below are suggested steps for setting daily priorities.

Steps for Setting Daily Priorities

Step 1. Make initial quick rounds on your patients, briefly checking the "big picture" of how they are doing before you go to report or sit down to study the plan of care. **Rationale:** This helps you identify problems requiring immediate attention and helps you connect the actual patients with what you hear during report or read in patient records.

Step 2. Immediately after shift report, verify critical information such as IV infusions, operation of equipment, and so forth. **Rationale:** Verifying information you received during report prevents misunderstandings and helps you and the nurse who's leaving settle problems while both of you are available for clarification.

Step 3. Identify urgent problems (those posing a significant immediate threat to the patient (eg, chest pain or a disconnected IV) and take appropriate action (eg, get help if needed). **Rationale:** Setting the wheels in motion to correct severe problems takes priority over taking time to analyze all the patient's problems.

Step 4. List the problems, including nursing diagnoses and collaborative problems, and ask the following questions:

What problems must be resolved today, and what happens if I wait until later?

What are the problems that I must monitor today, and what could happen if I don't monitor them?

To achieve the overall outcomes of care, what are the key problems that I must resolve, reduce, or control today?

Which of the patient's problems can I realistically work on today? **Rationale:** You can only do so much in a day. Answering the above questions helps you decide what *must* be done today.

Step 5. Determine the interventions that must be done to prevent, resolve, or control the problems listed. List these interventions along with routine tasks, such as baths, meals, and so forth. **Rationale:** This helps you get a big picture of the tasks of the day, which helps you answer questions such as, "What must be done first?" and "How can I make the best use of my time?" For example, you may give a routine bath to promote hygiene and, at the same time, discuss problems with coping.

Step 6. Decide what things the patient and his significant others can do on their own, what things to delegate to licensed practical nurses or unlicensed assistive personnel (UAP), and what things you must do personally (See Displays 5–1 and 5–2.) **Rationale:** The patient (and significant others) should be included in determining when things will get done and encouraged to be as independent as possible. Using less qualified workers appropriately allows you to spend more time accomplishing tasks that require the expertise of a registered nurse.

Step 7. Make a detailed personal worksheet for getting things done for the day, and refer to it frequently. Be sure to consider the daily routine of the unit (eg, when meals are served). **Rationale:** You're likely to experience many distractions during the course of the day. Don't rely on memory. Although the daily routine of the unit shouldn't dictate your activities, it's vital to consider when setting the schedule. Almost every nurse and many patients can recount stories of frustration caused by meals arriving during baths or the patient being called to physical therapy at inconvenient times.

Think About It

As the nurse, you're accountable for decisions made by UAPs. For example, in one case a nursing assistant caring for a young boy who was on a suicide watch told the nurse she was going on a break, leaving the child in the care of his mother. The mother left the room to go to the bathroom, and the child slipped away. Although the child was later found unharmed, the nurse would have been accountable for any injury incurred.

Assessing and Reassessing

Assessing patient status before interventions and then reassessing to monitor the *response* provides key information about the appropriateness of the plan of care: How is the patient responding? Are you getting the expected outcome? If not, why not? Do you need to make changes in the plan?

All too often today, your time for direct patient care is limited. Make it a habit to use every patient encounter as an opportunity to monitor physical and mental health status. For example, if you're helping someone bathe, you have the opportunity to assess skin status (by observing the entire body)) and mental status (by using therapeutic communication techniques). Remember to assess with an open mind. It's very easy to be misled by others' opinions. Consider the example on p. 159:

DISPLAY 5-1 Key Points of Delegation

Delegation defined: The transfer of responsibility for the performance of an activity while retaining accountability (ANA, 1995)

- **Remember the "four rights of delegation."*** (Hansten and Washburn, 1992)
  Delegate:
  1. **The right task** (one that can be delegated, rather than falling within nursing's scope of practice alone).
  2. **To the right person** (one qualified and competent to do the job).
  3. **Using the right communication** (clear, concise description of the task, the objective, and what you want reported).
  4. **Performing the right evaluation** (timely evaluation of the patient's response and worker's performance as the task is done and after the task is completed).
- **When should you delegate?**
  See Display 5–2.
- **What tasks should you delegate?**
  Tasks that are within the worker's job description (may be total tasks, such as taking vital signs, or partial tasks such as gathering equipment for a sterile dressing change).
- **How should you delegate?**
  With full knowledge of:
  - ✓ State nurse practice acts, standards, and policies and procedures (eg, A policy may state "RN is accountable for task completion and determining the degree of supervision appropriate to the AP and particular task").
  - ✓ Worker's capabilities and limitations.
  - ✓ The "four rights" of delegation.

Source: R. Alfaro-LeFevre Workshop handouts © 1996.

DISPLAY 5-2 When Should You Delegate?

Delegate	Don't Delegate
When the patient is stable	When complex assessment, thinking, and judgment are required
When task is within the worker's job description	When the outcome of the task is unpredictable
When the amount of RN time with the patient isn't significantly reduced	When there's increased risk of harm (eg, taking blood from an artery can incur more severe complications than venipuncture).
	When problem solving and creativity are required

Source: R. Alfaro-LeFevre workshop handouts © 1996.

EXAMPLE

> During report, Jodi, the evening nurse, was told that Mrs. French seemed to be somewhat "difficult" ("she doesn't want to ambulate or do anything").
>
> That evening, when Jodi went in to give Mrs. French her medications, she mentioned to her that she seemed very tired. Next, she asked if there was something that was causing her to feel this way. Mrs. French responded by explaining she hadn't slept well in weeks because she had just found out her daughter had breast cancer and was afraid she might die. This was important information that hadn't been offered before. Jodi was then able to talk with Mrs. French about her fears and concerns and offer a positive outlook by explaining that breast cancer, when detected early, has a good prognosis. By later that evening, Mrs. French was ambulating and talking about how eager she was to get home to some normalcy.
>
> Jodi was rewarded for her concern when she went into the room at midnight with a flash light to check Mrs. French's roommate's IV. Out of the darkness, she heard Mrs. French say, "Nurse?". Jodi responded, "Yes?". Then she heard Mrs. French whisper, "Thank you."

The above situation exemplifies the importance of performing ongoing data collection with an open mind while performing routine interventions.

Performing Nursing Interventions

Performing nursing interventions involves getting prepared, performing the interventions, monitoring the response, and making necessary changes.

Preparing to Act

Preparation can make the difference between risky, haphazard care that taxes both you and the person, and efficient, safe care that promotes comfort and gets results. Before you perform an intervention, prepare to act: be sure you know what you're going to do, why you're going to do it, how you're going to do it, and how you'll reduce risks of harm.

Steps for Preparing to Act

1. Review the plan and be sure you know the rationale and principles behind the intervention. If you don't know the principles and rationale, you won't be able to adapt the procedure if necessary, and you may not even recognize if the intervention is no longer appropriate.
2. Decide whether you have the qualifications (knowledge, skills, and authority) to perform the interventions.
3. Find out if the facility has procedures, protocols, guidelines, or standards that address how you should perform the interventions.
4. Assess the patient's *current status* and decide whether the interventions are still appropriate (compare your patient's situation with the plan of care).
5. Predict possible outcomes: Get a picture of what you're going to do, think about what might come up, what could go wrong, and what you'll do about it.

Weigh risks and benefits (page 135).

Identify ways to reduce risks of harm to the patient.

Identify ways to reduce the risks of harm to yourself.

Determine how to promote comfort and reduce patient stress (eg, if someone is expected to sit for a long period of time, get a comfortable chair and offer distractions).

6. Obtain the necessary resources (eg, equipment, personnel) and make sure you planned enough time and an environment conducive to performing the interventions.
7. Involve the person and significant others. Explain what's to be done and why, and how long it will take; encourage them to voice questions, suggestions, or concerns.

Think About It

The importance of assessment during Implementation *cannot be overemphasized. In fact, assessment errors are involved in most malpractice cases against nurses. For example, in one case, a 4-year-old child had to have emergency surgery to relieve pressure on blood vessels, nerves, and muscles caused by compartment syndrome (severe tissue swelling) after hip surgery. The nurses and hospital were found negligent. Evidence presented at the trial showed that the nurses hadn't monitored the child's condition appropriately. The fact that the nurses hadn't identified their own learning needs contributed to their negligence. They were held accountable for not knowing the equipment required to test for compartment syndrome and for not knowing where the equipment was located (Pirkov-Middaugh v Gillette Children's Hospital, 1991).*

Carrying Out Interventions and Making Necessary Changes

Once you've prepared to act, you're ready to carry out the actions. If you're prepared, your actions are likely to achieve the desired response. But what do you do if you don't get the desired response, the problem shows no improvement, or the situation is aggravated by the intervention?

If you don't get the desired response, a red flag that says something is wrong should go up in your mind. Stop and ask some key questions:

1. Did I perform the intervention(s) correctly?
2. Is the diagnosis correct, or has the problem or its cause changed? For example, suppose you were caring for someone with tachycardia, and the tachycardia didn't respond to cardiac medications. Your next question might be, "Could there be something else causing or contributing to the tachycardia (eg, anxiety, hypovolemia, respiratory problems)?".
3. Are there other interventions that would complement this intervention, increasing its effectiveness? For example, a backrub and talking with someone who's anxious is likely to enhance the effect of an anti-anxiety agent.
4. Could I be missing something? Should I be getting a second opinion?

Remember the following rule:

RULE ➧

> Always carry out nursing actions with full understanding of the principles and rationales involved, *closely observing the response*. If you don't get the desired response, start asking questions to find out what's wrong before continuing to act. When you find out what's wrong, make the necessary changes and record them on the plan of care as needed.

Case Management: Critical Paths and Variances in Care

If you're using a critical path like the one on page 240 to guide your patient's care, it sets priorities for you on a day-by-day basis—that is, *unless you identify a variance in care*. A *variance in care* occurs when a patient hasn't achieved outcomes by the timeframe noted on a critical path. For example, you've identified a variance in care if the critical path states "by the second day after surgery, the patient will be out of bed in a chair three times a day," but your patient isn't well enough to be out of bed three times a day.

What do you do if you identify a variance in care? Variance in care should trigger you to perform additional assessment to determine whether the delay is justified or whether actions need to be taken to improve the likelihood of achieving the outcome. Assessing for care variances by comparing your patient's *actual situation* to the critical path is crucial for safe and effective nursing care. Remember the following rule.

RULE ➧

> **Critical Thinking.** When using critical paths, never assume your patient is ready to progress as planned—*look* for care variances. If you identify a care variance, consider whether you need to contact a case manager for additional assessment and treatment.

Ethical/Legal Concerns

You're responsible, both legally and ethically, for protecting the client's right to privacy. This means you keep patient comments and information to yourself, and you limit access to patient records to those involved in the patient's care (students in an approved program may also have access for learning needs).

Ethically (and in some cases legally), you're responsible for *emotional* outcomes of your interventions as well as *physical* outcomes. For example, in some states, it's against the law to tell people they have AIDS over the phone. You must tell them in person and provide counseling and support. Here's another example: Suppose you plan to give someone who's having a facial tumor removed a pamphlet with graphic pictures of reconstructive surgery. As a prudent nurse, you must anticipate his response, stay with him, and provide support.

PRACTICE SESSION XV

Delegating, Case Management, Critical Paths, and Care Variances

To complete this session, read pages 154–161. Example responses can be found on page 235.

1. Suppose one of the many tasks that had to be accomplished today was getting a 30-year-old woman who has had a routine cholecystectomy out of bed for the first time:
   a. Would you delegate this task?
   no
   b. Why or why not?
   donot know response
2. Read "Think About It" on page 157.
   a. Why do you think the nurse is accountable for the child slipping away? (One to two sentences.)
   She knew aide was on break → therefore she was liable
   b. What could the nurse have done to decrease the likelihood of the child slipping away? (One to two sentences.)
   told mother not to leave had someone else watch him if she couldn't
3. Answer each letter below, using three to five sentences.
   a. How do you assess a patient for a care variance?
   You perform a complete assessment and determine whether pt is progressing
   b. What would you do if you identified a care variance and why?
   perform additional assessment to determine whether actions needed to be taken
   c. What can happen to the *patient* if you miss the fact that your patient is demonstrating a care variance?
   d. What can happen to *you* if you miss the fact that your patient is demonstrating a care variance?

Charting

Once you've given nursing care and evaluated the response, the next thing on your mind should be charting the assessments, interventions, and responses. Two reasons for this are:

1. You're likely to be more accurate and thorough if your memory is fresh.
2. Writing down what you've observed and done often jogs your memory about something *else* you need to assess or do. For example, you may be charting an abdominal assessment and realize you forgot to check to make sure the nasogastric tube suction equipment is functioning properly.

Keep in mind that the purpose of your charting is to:

1. Communicate care to other health care professionals who need to be able to find out what you've done and how the person is doing.
2. Help identify patterns of responses and changes in status.
3. Provide a foundation for evaluation, research, and improvement of the quality of care.
4. Create a legal document that may later be used in court to evaluate the type of care rendered. Your records can be your best friend or worst enemy. The best defense that you actually observed or did something is the fact that you made a note of it.
5. Supply validation for insurance purposes. The saying goes, "If it's not documented, they won't pay."

Different Ways of Charting

Different facilities often chart in different ways, combining one or more methods to meet their documentation goals. For this reason, it's a good idea to become familiar with all of the following charting methods:

Source-oriented charting: Caregivers from each discipline (medicine, nursing, physical therapy) chart on separate sheets, writing narrative notes chronologically. For an example, see Figure 5–2 on next page.

Focus charting®: Nurses use key words to organize charting (data, action, response), and the subject of the note isn't necessarily a problem (eg, may simply address a change in patient behavior). For an example, see Figure 5–3 on page 165.

Multidisciplinary charting: Caregivers from all disciplines write on the same record. For an example, see Figure 5–4 on page 166.

Flowsheet charting: These types of records cue you to chart specific information in specific spaces. If there's significant information to chart, you write in the allocated space; if there's no significant information to record, you place a check mark or dash in the space. Additional marks, such as an asterisk, may also be used to reflect when other pertinent information has been recorded somewhere else, such as on the medication record. For an example of flowsheet charting, see Figure 5–5 on page 157.

Date and Time	Problems and Diagnoses	Nursing Assessments and Comments
5/8/94 0800	*#1 Risk for Ineffective Airway Clearance related to thick secretions* *#2 Risk for Fluid Volume Deficit related to poor fluid intake*	Coughing up thick white mucus. He does this well, but needs to be reminded to work at it. Lungs have a few scattered rhonchi at both bases. Fluids encouraged, he does drink juices well. Apple juice on ice kept at bedside. ______ H. Laird, RN
1000		OOB to chair for 1/2 hour. States he feels very fatigued, but he is steady on his feet. Voided lge amount clear yellow urine. Allowed to rest before pulmonary function test. ______ H. Laird, RN
1100		To special studies via wheelchair for pulmonary function. ______ H. Laird, RN
1230		Returned via wheelchair. Assisted back to bed. Ate all of his lunch; said it was the first time he's been hungry. ______ H. Laird, RN

Figure **5–2.** Example of source-oriented narrative nurse's notes.

Charting by exception (CBE): Nurses refer to unit standards, policies, and protocols in the patient record, charting narrative notes only when the patient's data changes or care deviates from the norm. For an example, see Figure 5–6 on page 168.*

Use of addendum sheets: Nurses' notes are supplemented by separate sheets for each type of situation (eg, discharge summary sheets, teaching sheets). For an example, see Figure 5–7 on page 169.

Computerized patient records (CPR): Nursing notes are charted via computers. Use of CPR aims to eliminate repetitive charting and increase data base access. For an example, see Figure 5–8 on page 170.

Principles of Effective Charting

Effective charting must clearly show evidence of the following:

Initial assessments and reassessments: What did you observe when you first encountered the patient and at subsequent encounters, especially before and after interventions?

Status of client problems: What signs and symptoms do you observe in the person?

Interventions and nursing care performed: What did you do to meet the person's needs?

The response or outcomes of care: What results did you observe?

The person's ability to manage care needs after discharge: What did you observe that tells you the person will be able to manage care at home?

Display 5–3 on page 171 summarizes the criteria for effective charting systems.

---

*Recommended Reading: Burke, L., & Murphy, J. (1988). Charting by exception: A cost-effective, quality approach. New York: John Wiley & Sons.

Date	Focus	Progress Notes
5/8		
07:00	Wound care	D—States he's changed his mind about having wife do wound care at home. Says he wants to be self-sufficient and do own wound care.
		A—Encouraged him to view wound care video today.
		R—Requested to view video after AM care.
		R. Alfaro, RN

Figure **5–3.** Example of Focus Charting, using DAR to stand for data, action, response.

Learning to Chart Effectively

Learning to chart effectively requires knowledge and experience. As you improve your ability to assess people and discriminate between normal and abnormal findings, your charting will improve.

You can also improve your charting by practice and example.

1. Practice using the specific charting methods you'll be using before you go to the clinical setting.
2. Read charts to learn from actual situations. As you read the charts, ask yourself questions like "What are the diagnoses?", "Where's the evidence that the diagnoses exist?", "What are they doing to treat them?", and "How is this person responding?"

Although charting varies from place to place, there are some universal guidelines that apply to all charting. Take a few moments to review page 68 in Chapter 2, which lists guidelines for charting the initial data base, then go on to read the following guidelines.

Guidelines: Charting During Implementation

- Chart as soon as possible after giving nursing care. If you can't get to the chart, jot down notes on a worksheet. Don't rely on memory.
- Follow each facility's charting policies and procedures.
- Record important actions (eg, medication administration) immediately to be sure others know the action has been completed.
- Always record variations from the norm (eg, abnormalities in respiration, circulation, mental status, or behavior) and any actions taken related to the abnormalities (eg, if you reported the abnormality or if you intervened in some way).

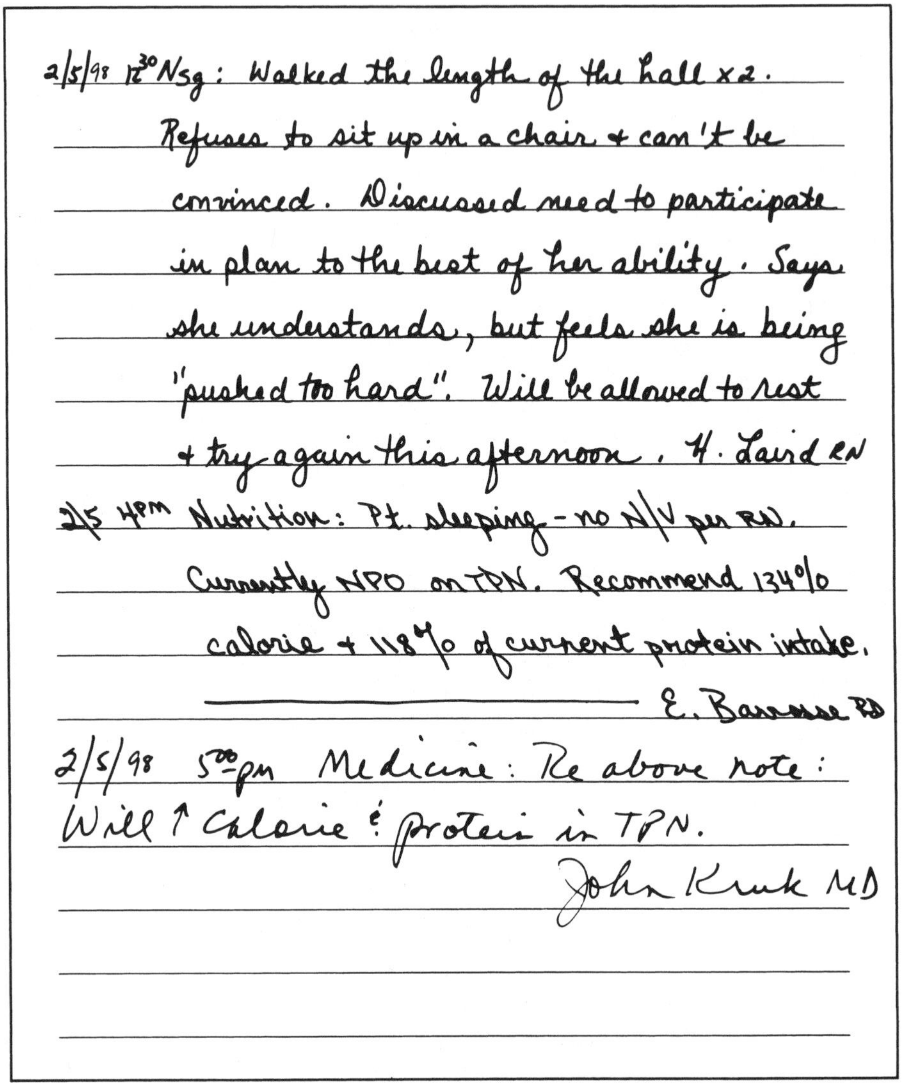

2/5/98 12³⁰ Nsg: Walked the length of the hall x2. Refuses to sit up in a chair + can't be convinced. Discussed need to participate in plan to the best of her ability. Says she understands, but feels she is being "pushed too hard". Will be allowed to rest + try again this afternoon. H. Laird RN

2/5 4PM Nutrition: Pt. sleeping - no N/V per RN. Currently NPO on TPN. Recommend 134% calorie + 118% of current protein intake. ———— E. Barrese RD

2/5/98 5⁰⁰ pm Medicine: Re above note: Will ↑ Calorie & protein in TPN. John Kruk MD

Figure 5–4. Example of multidisciplinary charting.

- Be precise. Your notes should provide a description and timeline for sequence of events, answering the questions *what happened* and *when, how, and where it happened.*

EXAMPLE

4/29/98 9:10 AM. Ambulated for 15 min to the end of the hall and back with wife's assistance. Gait is steady. Says he's "feeling stronger."

(text continued on page 173)

© 1985
St. Luke's Hospital
Milwaukee, Wisconsin

NURSING/PHYSICIAN
ORDER FLOWSHEET
05-937555 Rev. 12/85

Date 6/3 - 6/4

Karl Stitt

NRSG DX	NURSING/PHYSICIAN ORDER												
1	Neurologic assessment – include short term memory	08 *	09 *	930 *	2000 *	2100 *	2230 *	01 *	04 →	06 →			
1	Neurovascular assessment	08 *	09 *	930 *	2000 *	2100 *	2230 *	01 *	04 →	06 →			
1	Tolerance of ADL's	08 ✓	09 ✓										
1	Signs + Symptoms of Bldg	08 ✓	16 ✓										
*	NURSE INITIAL ▶ SIGNIFICANT FINDINGS ▼	LB	GS	GS	GS	GS	GS	JB	JB	JB			

NRSG DX#	TIME		INIT
1	0800	® arm still feels heavy, speech slow but pt states he feels he's improving every day. Needs minimal assistance c̄ ADLs. Is able to set up his own tray and do own bath with assistance when chair is placed in bathroom. Ambulated to nurses station with 1 person standby assist. —	LB
1	1600	c/o mild blurred vision & ® hand numbness.	GS.
1	1900	States he feels worse, like when he was first admitted. c/o ® hand feeling "like it was dead". Weak ® hand grasp, much diminished from ® arm. Has very slow slurred speech, difficulty forming words. Dr Ferguson notified. Immediately came up to see pt. Orders written. Wife called by nurse. Notified of change in pt. status. —	GS
1	2030	Speech improving. ® hand numbness decreasing —	GS.
1	2130	Unable to speak. Able to communicate through head nods + gestures. No ® arm grasp. Dr Ferguson called. No new orders.	
1	2230	Able to speak, but talks slowly. Has difficulty forming words. c/o "funny feeling" on ® arm, but couldn't be more specific. States feeling went away in 5 minutes. Able to lift arm in full ROM. Strong Ⓛ hand grasp. ® hand grasp < Ⓛ. States ® hand numbness is decreasing.	GS.

INIT	R.N. SIGNATURE	INIT	R.N. SIGNATURE	INIT	R.N. SIGNATURE
LB	Lorraine Buhler RN	JB	Joan Bishop RN		
GS	Glenda Schuster RN	JK	Jackie Kruck RN		

➜ See Reverse Side NURSING/PHYSICIAN ORDER FLOW SHEET Dist. White-Chart Yellow-Bedside

Figure 5–5. Example of flowsheet charting. (From Burke, L. & Murphy, J. [1988]. *Charting by exception* [p.123]. New York: John Wiley & Sons.)

ASSESSMENT PARAMETERS

The following parameters will be considered a negative assessment. If the physical assessment is negative indicate with a "✓" followed by initials in the box after the particular assessment area. An asterisk (*) followed by initials in the box is to be used to chart the exceptions which require elaboration in the box to the right.

Head Assessment:

Fontanelles level; soft. Sutures approximated. No infections, lice, alopecia, scabies or crusting. No headache

Integumentary Assessment

Skin warm, dry and intact. Turgor elastic. No lesions, masses, lacerations, bruises or rashes. Mucous membranes moist and pink.

EENT Assessment

Vision clear with or without glasses. Responds to spoken voice. Tm's pearly; ext. canals clear, nares patent, moist, and no discharge. Mouth and throat without lesions, erythema or exudate, tonsils 1-2+. Neck supple. Trachea midline, able to make swallowing movements. No lymphadenopathy.

Respiratory Assessment *See reverse side for respiratory rates

Resps quiet and regular. Rate within normal limits for age. No flaring or retractions. Breath sounds vesicular through both lung fields, bronchial over major airways with no adventitious sounds, no cough.

Cardiovascular Assessment *See reverse side for heart rates

Regular apical pulse and rate within limits for age. No extra heart sounds. Peripheral pulses palpable bil. No edema. No cyanosis of circumoral areas or nail beds. Capillary refill brisk.

Gasrointestinal Assessment

Abdomen soft. Bowel sounds active all 4 quadrants. No pain with palpation. No abnormal movements. Tolerates prescribed diet without nausea & vomiting. Having BM's within normal pattern and consistency.

TEMPERATURE (one only) ˚C			PULSE	RESP	INIT	NURSE SIGNATURE	DATE	TIME
A	O	R	AP	R				
BLOOD PRESSURE ☐ MANUAL ☐ MONITOR ____ Cuff Size								
RECUMBENT BP RT LEFT		SITTING BP RT LEFT		STANDING BP RT LEFT				
WEIGHT ____ kg ☐ standing Hc ____ cms ____ lbs ☐ infant scale chest ____ cms				HEIGHT ____ cms ____ ins				

Figure 5–6. Sample of pediatric nursing data base using normal assessment parameters and charting by exception. (Courtesy Memorial Hospital at Easton, Md.)

ANTICOAGULANT

Karl Stitt

KNOWLEDGE OR SKILL CRITERIA* TO BE MET BEFORE DISCHARGE BY THE ( ) PATIENT ( ) SPOUSE OR SIGNIFICANT OTHER:	TEACHING AND/OR REINFORCEMENT (DATE/INITIALS)				MEETS CRITERIA (DATE/INITIALS)
1. Verbalizes basic Coumadin pharmacology (purpose, action, dosage)	6/4	GS			6/5 LB
2. Verbalizes possible major side effects.	6/4	GS			6/5 LB
3. Verbalizes time, date, and place of scheduled post-discharge Prothrombin Time tests and to check with M.D. for results.	6/6	GS			6/5 LB
4. Verbalizes importance of adherence to medication regimen and results of omission (thrombi, emboli, phlebitis).	6/6	GS			6/7 LB
5. Verbalizes precautionary measures to be taken while on Coumadin therapy:					
a. take only meds per M.D. order (no ASA meds)	6/5	LB			6/6 GS
b. aware of meds that alter Coumadin actions (BCPs, vitamins, hormones)	6/5	LB			6/6 GS
c. carry ID card or medic alert jewelry	6/6	LB			6/7 LB
d. prevent physical injury when possible (shave with electric shaver, do not go barefoot, etc.)	6/6	LB			6/7 LB
6. Verbalizes appropriate action if persistent bleeding occurs.	6/6	GS			6/7 LB
7. Verbalizes need to inform all M.D.s. and dentists of anticoagulant therapy.	6/6	GS			6/7 LB

*SEE NURSE'S DISCHARGE NOTE FOR DOCUMENTATION ON TEACHING RE: ADL RESTRICTIONS, DIETARY CHANGES, MEDICATIONS, TREATMENTS, OR FOLLOW-UP MEDICAL CARE. 6/3 Hard of hearing (both ears) LB

SPECIAL LEARNING NEEDS:

TEACHING RESOURCES UTILIZED	DATE	INITIALS	TEACHING RESOURCES UTILIZED	DATE	INITIALS
Coumadin Medication Sheet (330-05)			Anticoagulant teaching sheet.	6/8	LB
MedicAlert Jewelry Information	6/6	GS			
ID Card for Anticoagulant Therapy	6/8	LB			

SIGNATURE	INITIALS	SIGNATURE	INITIALS	SIGNATURE	INITIALS
Lorraine Buhler RN	LB				
Glenda Schuster RN	GS				

ST. LUKE'S HOSPITAL, MILWAUKEE WI — PATIENT TEACHING RECORD — 8/80; REV. 12/86, 5/87 X-12C

Figure 5–7. Sample addendum sheet for teaching. (From Burke, L. & Murphy, J. [1988]. *Charting by exception* [p.127]. New York: John Wiley & Sons.)

NAME: JANE DOE FT NO: ADM PHYS: D. HOWSER
ADM DX: PNEUMONIA/CHF AGE: 69 ROOM/BED: 0304-02
MEDICAL RECORD NUMBER: SEX: F ADM DATE: 01/23/94

CARE FACTORS ASSIGNED	TIME	ASSESSMENT/REASSESSMENT/EXCEPTION
ONGOING REASSESSMENT		
BSC/BRF WITH ASSIST	8:30	Resp ↑ 36 c̄ rales ½ way ↑ on Ⓡ and
CATHETER CARE		¼ ↑ on Ⓛ. Dr DeMarino notified. O_2 placed
EMOTIONAL SUPPORT		on @ 35% via mask. Lasix 80mg
REVIEW/EVALUATE/DOCUMENT CARE		given IV. Resting in semi fowlers.
COMPLETE BATH BY PERSONNEL	930	Diuresing cl. yellow urine
TURNING AND SKIN CARE		Breathing better (↓32/min) + less
INDIRECT CARE, 3 WEST		labored. Coughing up thick yellow
(PO), GTTS, PR, (OINT) OR MEDS BY NGT		mucus. Alert — taking
IVPB/ANY NUMBER		liquids well.
CON'T IV-SITE ASSESSED Q SHIFT	1030	Lungs much improved - still
TITRATED MEDS/PCA		have rales at both bases, but
DOB TO CHAIR 1 (2) ASS'T TID		R↓26/min. Assisted OOB to
FEEDS WITH ASS'T		chair — tolerated well.
BLOOD GLUCOSE MONITORING	1430	Resting — respirations non-
INTAKE AND OUTPUT		labored. C. Keggler RN
FALL PREVENTION PROGRAM		
*REVIEW/REVISE/UPDATE CARE PLAN		
*OXYGEN ADMINISTRATION		
FREQUENT SUCTIONING-ORAL/TRAC		
VS ROUTINE TO Q4H		
CARDIAC MONITORING & INTERPRET		
D/C'D		
Daily Weights x 1 week		

ENTER ADDITIONAL COMMENTS ON BACK

CLASSIFICATION BY: HOURS: STANDARD OF CARE/PRACTICE. FOLLOWED/EXCEPTIONS NOTED.

SHIFT: SIGNATURES:

MULTIDISCIPLINARY COLLABORATION WITH:

DISCHARGE PLANNING	(✓)	DIETARY	( )	8-4	C. Keggler RN
HOME CARE	( )	CPT	( )	4-12	M. Riley RN
FT/OT	( )	OTHER	( )	12-8	C. Sechrist RN
CLERGY	( )	CHAPLIN	( )		

	INTAKE: ORAL	PARENTERAL	OTHER	TOTAL	OUTPUT: URINE	NG TUBE/EMESIS	DRAINS	OTHER	TOTAL
8-4	360	900		1260	400				400
4-12	480	650		1130	200				200
12-8	150	0		100	100				100
24 HR	990	1550		2540	700				700

Figure 5-8. Example of computer-assisted charting. (Patient care flowsheet from Paoli Memorial Hospital. Paoli, PA.)

DISPLAY 5-3 Criteria for Effective Charting Systems

Effective charting systems should

- Be tailor-made to the types of problems frequently demonstrated by the patient population of the facility, to direct nurses to chart key aspects of patient care.
- Reflect use of nursing process.
- Discourage double documentation (charting the same thing in two different places) and irrelevant charting.
- Increase the quality of nursing records, while reducing the amount of time spent charting.
- Be designed so crucial patient data (eg, assessments and interventions) are easily retrievable, thereby facilitating communication, evaluation, research, and quality improvement.
- Be legally sound.

- Use a mnemonic to organize your charting. (Display 5–4, which explains common mnemonics used for charting such as AIR-A, DAR, DIE.)
- Focus on significant problems or events that communicate *what's different* about this person today. For example, don't record, "went to the bathroom unassisted," unless this is unusual.
- Stick to the facts. Avoid judgmental language.

EXAMPLE

Right: "Shouting, 'Everyone had better stay away from me, or I'm likely to hit some-one.' "
Wrong: "Angry and aggressive."

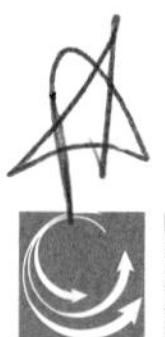

DISPLAY 5-4 Mnemonics Used for Charting

AIR-A (Assessment, Intervention, Response, Action). Chart the *assessment* data you observe, the *intervention(s)* performed, the patient's *response* to intervention(s), and any *action(s)* you took based on the response.
DAR (Data Action Response). Chart the *data* you observe, the *action*(s) performed, and the *response* of the patient.
DIE (Data, Intervention, Evaluation). Chart the *data* you observe, the *intervention(s)* performed, and your *evaluation* of the patient's response.
PIE (Problem, Interventions, Evaluation). Chart the status of the *problem(s)*, the *intervention(s)* performed, and the *evaluation* of the patient's response to the interventions.**SOAP, SOAPIE** See page 146.

- Be specific. Don't use vague terms.

EXAMPLE

> **Right:** Abdominal dressing has an area of light pink drainage about 6 inches in diameter.
> **Wrong:** Noted moderate amount of drainage on abdominal dressing.

- Be concise, yet descriptive. You don't have to write complete sentences, but use adjectives and accepted abbreviations to give a good picture of activities and observations.

EXAMPLE

> **Right:** OOB to chair for a half hour—no side effects.
> **Wrong:** OOB to chair for a half hour. Seems to have tolerated it well because no obvious side effects were noted.

- Sign your name consistently, using your first initial, last name, and credentials after each entry that you complete (eg, F. Nightingale, RN).
- Never leave a blank line; draw a line through unused spaces before and after your signature. (Note the example in Fig. 5–2.)
- When you forget to chart something, record it as soon as you can, marking it a late entry.

EXAMPLE

> 5/17/98 3:00 PM, Late entry: Stool was positive for blood at 10 AM this morning. Notified Dr. Eyler. R. Alfaro-LeFevre, RN.

- Record failure or refusal to follow prescribed regimen, as well as any actions taken.

EXAMPLE

> Refuses to go to physical therapy. Says it "doesn't do any good." Notified Dr. Frazier and Rochelle Hutton in physical therapy.

PRACTICE SESSION XVI

Principles of Effective Charting

To complete this session, read pages 163–172. Example responses can be found on page 236. You may either write or tape-record your responses, if appropriate.

1. List five functions that patient records serve.

① Communicate care to other health care prof.
② Help identify changes in pattern of response and status
③ Provide a foundation for evaluation, research, improvement of quality care
④ Creates legal document - used in court
⑤ Supply validation for insurance purposes.

2. Give two reasons why you should chart as soon as possible after giving nursing care. -more accurate
-triggers you to remember what you've forgotten

3. Imagine a patient calls you into the room and tells you she feels like she's choking on mucus, but is afraid to cough because of abdominal incisional pain. You help her to get in a better position, and then assist her to splint the incision with a pillow. She finally coughs up a gray mucus plug and thanks you for your help. You listen to her lungs and they sound clear. You emphasize the importance of reporting incisional pain that interferes with breathing. Using the mnemonic DAR, AIR-A, or DIE, write a note that records the above event.

4. What's wrong with the following two excerpts from nurses' notes?

a. 5/8 Patient is difficult and uncooperative. R. Alfaro-LeFevre, RN.

b. 5/8 Patient seems confused. R. Alfaro-LeFevre, RN.

5. Pretend you wrote the nurse's note below on the wrong chart. Correct it using the accepted method for correcting charting errors.

5/8 N/G tube draining light green drainage.

Giving the Change-of-Shift Report

Your goal when giving report should be to give accurate, factual, organized information. What you say and how you say it can make a big difference in the quality of care your patient receives. For example, consider the two following reports, which present two versions of the same information.

Verbal Nursing Reports

Verbal Nursing Report 1

"Mrs. J. has had her usual bad day. She's driving me nuts with her moaning and groaning about her back pain. I've given her everything I can, but she's still on the light all the time . . . and she even has her husband hopping around for every little request! The x-rays have been negative. This has been going on for 2 weeks! I wish they'd do something with her. I think she's just a hypochondriac, and this isn't a psychiatric unit. Her signs are stable, and intake and output are okay. Good luck with her."

Verbal Nursing Report 2

"Mrs. J. seems to have had another bad day. She states the pain medicine gives very little relief, if any. Her husband has been very supportive and tries to help her, but nothing seems to work. The x-rays have been negative. It must be really hard to be here for 2 weeks without getting any better or finding out what's wrong. Her vital signs are stable and she's had 700 mL intake today. She should be encouraged to drink more during the evening."

Note the negativism and subjectivity of Report 1. The nurse has begun to pass on the word that "this patient is a hypochondriac." If continued, the attitude of the whole nursing staff can become negative. On the other hand, the nurse in Report 2 states the facts and offers an empathetic view of how Mrs. J. must be feeling.

The following guidelines are presented to help you establish good habits for giving report.

Guidelines: Giving Change-of-Shift Reports

- Use a written or printed guide to prompt you to be thorough and organized (eg, use a worksheet like the one on page 155, a flowsheet, or care plan).
- Begin by giving basic background information, including the following: name, room number, age, attending and consulting physicians, date of admission, medical diagnoses, surgical procedures, and nursing diagnoses.

EXAMPLE

> "Mrs. Ballard, in room 214 by the window, is a 35-year-old patient of Dr. Smith, with a consultation to Dr. Jones. She was admitted on 5/25 with pneumonia. She had a tracheostomy on 5/26. She has *Ineffective Airway Clearance related to thick and copious secretions.*

- Be specific. Avoid vague terms.

EXAMPLE

> **Right:** "Mrs. Wu has had an increase in her respiratory rate to 32/min. Her heart rate is up to 122, and her temperature is 101°F."
> **Wrong:** "Mrs. Wu seems to be having respiratory difficulty."
> **Right:** "I gave Mrs. Wu 8 mg of morphine IM at 5:10 PM for incisional pain."
> **Wrong:** "I gave Mrs. Wu a pain med for her pain."

- If you make an inference, back it up with evidence.
- Describe the presence of all invasive treatments (eg, intravenous lines, Foley catheters, nasogastric tubes).
- Stress abnormal findings (eg, rales in the lungs, abnormal vital signs) and variations from routine or the norm (eg, "This patient *won't* have a preop medication.")

Ongoing Evaluation

Although how to conduct a complete formal evaluation is addressed in depth in Chapter 6, remember that a key activity of *Implementation* is *ongoing evaluation.* You're responsible for monitoring progress and updating the plan as needed even before you get to a formal evaluation. Display 5–5 shows the type of questions you should be asking to make sure the plan of care is kept up to date during *Implementation.*

It's also important to perform early evaluation of how *your* days are going, looking for ways to improve your performance and satisfaction with your job. Display 5–6 lists questions to ask yourself to evaluate your workday.

DISPLAY 5–5 Questions to Ask to Determine if the Plan of Care is Up to Date

- Does your patient still exhibit the problems identified on the plan?
- Are there problems your patient has that *aren't* addressed on the plan of care, but may impede progress to outcome achievement?
- Are the expected outcomes still realistic?
- Are the interventions still relevant?

DISPLAY 5–6 Questions to Ask Yourself to Critique Your Work Day

- How has the day gone in general?
- Have I completed everything I should have?
- Have I been able to set priorities well?
- Have I been organized?
- What are the factors that have influenced how I set priorities and organized my day?
- Have I been clear and specific when delegating actions?
- How much time am I spending performing collaborative nursing interventions?
- How much time am I spending implementing independent nursing interventions?
- Could I be doing more?
- Am I trying to do too much?
- What changes should I make tomorrow?

Summary

Implementation requires you to put the plan into action with an active, open mind—a mind that's constantly assessing and reassessing both patient responses and your own performance. People are unpredictable. Monitor them carefully and be willing to be flexible and change approaches as needed on a day-to-day (even hour-to-hour) basis. With today's reduced length of stays, and increased use of UAPs, use every patient encounter as an opportunity to observe mental and physical status. Be sure you know how to delegate effectively (page 158). Also work to become competent in communicating patient care (charting and reporting), setting priorities, and delegating tasks effectively.

Evaluate your knowledge of this chapter. Check to see if you can achieve the objectives on page 152.

Bibliography: See pages 189–191.

CHAPTER 6

Evaluation

OBJECTIVES

Once you complete this chapter, you should be able to:

- Explain how to determine outcome achievement.
- Discuss how to decide whether to terminate, continue, or modify the plan of care.
- Describe the steps involved in evaluation of an individual plan of care.
- Explain why it's important to perform all three types of evaluation studies—outcome, process, and structure—to improve care quality.
- Describe the staff nurse's role in relation to quality improvement (QI).

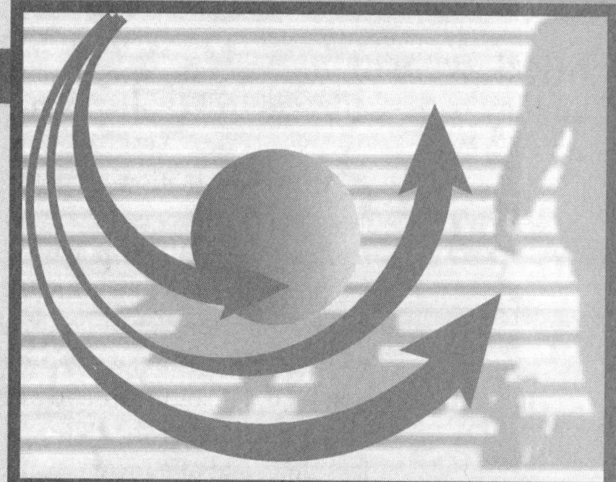

Standard V: *Evaluation.* The nurse evaluates the client's progress toward attainment of outcomes.*

Practice Sessions

- **Practice Session XVII:** Determining Outcome Achievement, Identifying Variables Affecting Outcome Achievement, and Deciding Whether to Continue, Modify, or Terminate the Plan
- **Practice Session XVIII:** Quality Improvement

What's in this chapter?

Although the need for *ongoing* evaluation during *Implementation* was emphasized in Chapter 5, Chapter 6 focuses on how to perform a *formal* evaluation of an individual plan of care—that is, how to decide whether to continue, modify, or terminate the plan and discharge the person. It also addresses the importance of ongoing, systematic quality improvement (QI) studies to correct and improve health care delivery practices.

*Excerpted from ANA Standards of Clinical Nursing Practice (1991).

Critical Evaluation: The Key to Excellence in Health Care Delivery

Critical evaluation—careful, deliberate, and detailed evaluation of various aspects of patient care—is the key to excellence in health care delivery. It can make the difference between care practices that are doomed to repeat errors and care practices that are progressive, and constantly improving.

Most often you'll be involved in evaluating an individual plan of care. However, with increasing frequency, you're likely to be asked to help in another type of evaluation—QI. QI studies aim to evaluate *groups of patients* or specific *aspects of care* to improve care quality for all (eg, How can we achieve the same outcomes with less pain, in less time, and at a lower cost?).

First, let's look at what *Evaluation* entails in the context of an individual plan of care, then consider *Evaluation* in the context of QI.

Evaluation of an Individual Plan of Care

Evaluation of an individual plan includes:

- Determining outcome achievement.
- Identifying the variables (factors) affecting outcome achievement.
- Deciding whether to continue, modify, or terminate the plan.
- Continuing, modifying, or terminating the plan.

Determining Outcome Achievement

The following steps are suggested to evaluate outcome achievement.

Steps for Evaluating Outcome Achievement

1. Determine current health status and readiness to test for outcome achievement.
2. List the outcomes set forth in *Planning*.

EXAMPLE

> "Will walk unassisted the length of the hall by 7/3."

3. Compare what the person is able to do in relation to the outcomes.

EXAMPLE

> "Can walk unassisted the length of the hall, but becomes unsteady toward the end of the hall."

4. Decide the extent of outcome achievement by asking the following questions:
   Have the outcomes been completely met?
   Have the outcomes been partially met?
   Have the outcomes not at all been met?

5. Record your findings on the patient or client record (progress notes, plan of care).

Identifying Variables Affecting Outcome Achievement

Identifying the variables (factors) affecting outcome achievement requires analyzing information gained from assessing the patient and chart. You need to answer the following questions:

1. Were the outcomes and interventions realistic and appropriate for this individual?
2. Were the interventions implemented consistently as prescribed?
3. Were new problems or adverse responses detected early, and were appropriate changes made?
4. What's the person's opinion concerning outcome achievement and the plan of care?
5. What factors impeded progress?
6. What factors enhanced progress?
7. Was the literature searched for applicable research and practice articles?

Deciding Whether to Continue, Modify, or Terminate the Plan

The final step is deciding whether to continue, modify, or terminate the plan.

- **Continue the plan** if the person hasn't achieved outcomes, but you haven't identified any factors that impeded or enhanced care and simply require more time. (Keep in mind that people failing to achieve desired outcomes in the expected timeframe are demonstrating a *care variance,* which should be evaluated by a case manager.)
- **Modify the plan** when outcomes haven't been achieved, when you identify new problems or risk factors, or when you identify ways to make care more effective.
- **Terminate the plan** if the person has achieved outcomes, has no new problems or risk factors, and demonstrates ability to care for herself. Display 6–1 provides steps for terminating the plan.

DISPLAY 6–1 Steps For Terminating The Plan of Care

1. Determine how health care will be managed at home (see Display 4–6 for the types of questions to ask for discharge).
2. Give verbal and written instructions for:
   - Treatments, medications, activities, diet.
   - What signs and symptoms must be reported.
   - How to reach relevant community resources.
3. Once you've taught the patient and significant others the above information, ask them to repeat the information, using the written instructions, if necessary (instructions don't have to be *memorized*).
4. If the patient and significant others demonstrate knowledge of how to manage health care at home, discharge the patient according to facility policy.

Examining the Other Steps of the Nursing Process

The following illustration provides a visual summary of the process of evaluating an individual plan of care.

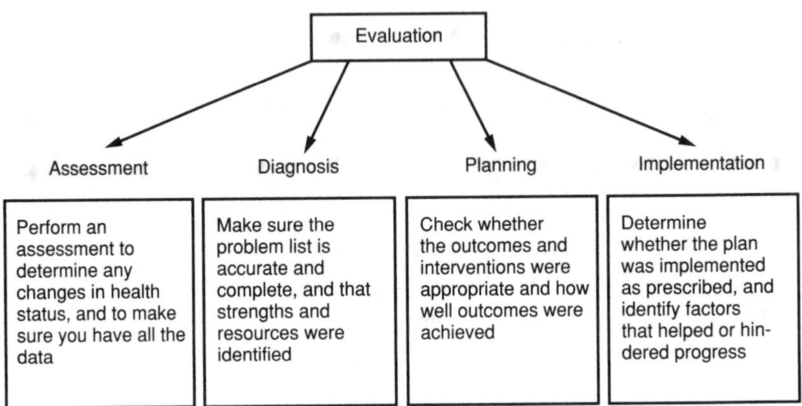
Evaluation
Assessment
Diagnosis
Planning
Implementation
Perform an assessment to determine any changes in health status, and to make sure you have all the data
Make sure the problem list is accurate and complete, and that strengths and resources were identified
Check whether the outcomes and interventions were appropriate and how well outcomes were achieved
Determine whether the plan was implemented as prescribed, and identify factors that helped or hindered progress

PRACTICE SESSION XVII

Determining Outcome Achievement, Identifying Variables Affecting Achievement, and Deciding Whether to Continue, Modify, or Terminate the Plan

To complete this session, read pages 180–182. Example responses can be found on page 236. You may either write or tape-record your responses, if appropriate.

Part I.

Outcome Achievement. For each number below, compare the outcome criteria with the listed observable patient data. Circle "A" if the outcome has been *achieved.* Circle "P" if the outcome has only been *partially* met. Circle "N" if the outcome has *not* been met.

1. **Outcome:** Will demonstrate self-injection of insulin using aseptic technique.
   Observable Data: Injected self using good technique, but contaminated needle without noticing it.
   Answer: A P N
2. **Outcome:** Will demonstrate safe crutch walking, including climbing and descending stairs.
   Observable Data: Demonstrates ability to use crutches for walking, climbing, and descending without problems.
   Answer: A P N
3. **Outcome:** Will relate the effect of increased exercise upon insulin demand.
   Observable Data: States that insulin demand is not affected by increased exercise.
   Answer: A P N

4. **Outcome:** Will maintain skin free from signs of irritation.
   Observable Data: Skin is intact, with some reddened areas noted on both elbows.
   Answer: A P N

5. **Outcome:** Will list the signs and symptoms of infection.
   Observable Data: Lists pain, swelling, and drainage.
   Answer: A P N

Part II.

How do you know whether to terminate, continue, or modify the plan?

Ongoing, Systematic Evaluation for Quality Improvement (QI)

The concept of QI is based on the philosophy that quality can almost always be improved—what is accepted as quality today may be substandard tomorrow, especially if you consider modern advances, such as diagnostic and treatment modalities, computers, and communication systems.

Almost every facility has a QI committee, whose charge is to examine and improve care by performing ongoing:

Literature searches for research and practice articles related to current care practices (eg, searching online each month for the latest pain management articles).

Systematic and focused evaluation of patient records. For example, consider the case study below, which shows the importance of identifying problems and finding solutions through QI studies.

CASE STUDY

A QI nurse was studying data about how long patients stayed in the hospital for certain problems. He noted that patients who came to his hospital with pneumonia stayed 1 day longer than patients with the same diagnosis in most hospitals. He recognized this to be a problem: Why did it take patients in his hospital 1 day longer to get well enough to go home? After an in-depth study of the records of all patients who were admitted with pneumonia in the previous 2 years, he identified a simple, but crucial, delay in health care delivery: antibiotics weren't coming from the pharmacy in a timely fashion. On the whole, patients in his hospital started on antibiotics 12 to 24 hours after admission (compared to within 4 hours at other hospitals). Based on this information, new policies were made to ensure that antibiotics and other important medications were delivered to patient units immediately, and given within 4 hours of admission. The problem with length of stay was resolved. ■

The above case shows how collecting and reviewing data about specific problems offers crucial insights into how well care management practices are working, and how they can be improved.

Three Types of Evaluation

To best monitor health care practices, QI studies should consider three types of evaluation:

Outcome Evaluation: Focuses on the *results, or outcomes* of care (eg, Were outcomes achieved? Are people satisfied with care?).

Process Evaluation: Focuses on *how the care was given* (eg, Were assessments and interventions performed consistently and in a timely manner?).

Structure Evaluation: Focuses on the *setting* in which the care takes place (eg, Were the physical environment, staffing patterns, and organization communication practices adequate for efficient care management?).

Considering all three types of evaluation—outcome, process, and structure—provides a comprehensive examination of care management. Display 6–2 shows example questions for all three types of studies.

Staff Nurses' Role

All staff nurses are accountable for participating in QI studies (most often for data collection and tracking outcomes). Although some of these QI studies may seem long and complicated, as the bedside nurse, you're in a unique position to make a valuable contribution to QI. Keep in mind the following:

- How you document is important. The records you create through ongoing documentation provide the basis for research that can benefit both health care consumers and nurses.
- QI studies may seem complicated and detailed, but they make your job more efficient and may make your (or your family's) next contact with the health care system more efficient.

DISPLAY 6–2 Examples of Questions to Ask for Three Types of QI Studies

Outcome Evaluation (focus on results): How many of our patients undergoing appendectomy experience an infection severe enough to delay discharge?
Process Evaluation (focus on how care was given): At what point was each of our patients undergoing appendectomy first given antibiotics?
Structure Evaluation (focus on setting): In what setting were antibiotics given to each of our patients undergoing appendectomy (eg, emergency department? operating room? medical-surgical floor?).

Source: R. Alfaro-LeFevre workshop handouts © 1996.

- Stay up-to-date with the terminology so you know why the studies are being done. (See Display 6–3 for explanation of terms related to QI.)
- Be willing to get involved. You are the one who spends the most time at the bedside; if you see human problems or problems with hospital policies or procedures, report them to your supervising nurse. If you're asked to do extra documentation for the purpose of these studies, realize that the information gained from the records is essential to improving quality.

Think About It

We can always improve. Most hospitals devise their own critical pathways after inviting representatives from several disciplines to work out an agreement on a plan of care. However, many seem to fall short in follow-up (eg, monitoring, evaluating, and updating their pathways). A survey showed that less than half of the respondents monitor the effects of pathways on variables such as complications, patient and family satisfaction, and use of resources. Collecting and reviewing these data is important because it offers crucial insights into how well patient care management practices are working. The survey, returned by 346 health care institutions for a 44% response rate revealed that at 33% of responding centers there was no ongoing review of and evaluation of critical pathways. (—. 1996. Critical Pathways Data Review Offers Crucial Insight. AACN News, *July, p. 5)*

DISPLAY 6–3 Definition and Discussion of Terms Related to Quality Improvement

Note: Although there are varying formal definitions of the following terms, these definitions are designed to be understandable for beginning nursing students.

Quality: The degree to which patient care services increase the probability of achieving *desired* outcomes with decreased probability of *undesired* outcomes.

Quality Assessment (QA): Ongoing studies designed to evaluate quality of patient care and services. *Discussion*. Just as *Assessment* is the first step of the nursing process, QA is the first step of QI.

Quality Improvement (QI): Ongoing studies designed to identify ways to promote achievement of desired outcomes in a timely, cost-effective fashion, while decreasing the risks for undesired outcomes. *Discussion*. QI studies may focus on identifying and correcting system problems (eg, ineffective policies and procedures, poor communication between departments, or duplication of services), or simply finding ways to "make things better" (even if no problem exists).

Continuous Quality Improvement (CQI): See QI above.

Persistent Quality Improvement (PQI): See QI above.

(continued)

DISPLAY 6–3 Definition and Discussion of Terms Related to Quality Improvement (Continued)

Performance Assessment and Improvement: Ongoing studies designed to improve quality of health care services by examining "nine dimensions of quality": acceptability, access, appropriateness, continuity, effectiveness, efficacy, efficiency, safety, and timeliness.
Total Quality Management (TQM): Management that focuses on promoting achievement of desirable outcomes with reduced risk of undesirable outcomes by making changes based on the results of quality improvement studies.
Indicator: Something that measures specific objective events or occurrences that provide information about the quality of care services. For example, in the case history on page 183, the indicator that might be examined to determine quality of care is the amount of time that elapsed from the time the patient was admitted to the time the patient began receiving antibiotics.

Summary

Critical evaluation—careful, deliberate, and detailed evaluation of various aspects of patient care—is the key to excellence in health care delivery. *Evaluation* in the context of nursing process usually refers to determining the effectiveness of an individual plan of care (ie, Did the patient achieve the outcomes in a timely manner?). Within the context of QI, *Evaluation* refers to ongoing studies of *groups of patients* to examine the effectiveness of care delivery practices. Comprehensive QI studies evaluate outcomes (results), process (how care was given), and structure (the setting in which care was given).

PRACTICE SESSION XVIII

Quality Improvement

To complete this session, read pages 183–186. Example responses can be found on page 236. You may either write or tape-record your responses. If appropriate

1. In 1 to 2 sentences or phrases, explain why quality improvement studies are important.

2. Why is it important to consider outcome, process, and structure when performing QI studies?

3. What do QI, CQI, and PQI have in common?

4. In 2 or 3 sentences, explain the staff nurse's responsibilities in relation to *QI*.

(1) Report areas of improvement
(2) Keep accurate records
(3) Applying results of QI studies to their practice

Evaluate your knowledge of this chapter. Check to see if you can achieve the objectives on page 178.

Bibliography: See pages 189–191.

Bibliography

———. (1996). Critical pathways data review offers crucial insight. *AACN News,* July, p. 2.

Aiken, T., & Catalano, J. (1994). *Legal, ethical and political issues in nursing*. Philadelphia: Davis.

Alfaro-LeFevre, R. (1995). *Critical thinking in nursing: A practical approach.* Philadelphia: W.B. Saunders.

Alfaro-LeFevre, R. (1996). *Instructor's manual for critical thinking in nursing: A practical approach.* Philadelphia: W.B. Saunders.

American Association of Critical Care Nurses (1995). *Delegation: A tool for success in the changing workplace.* AACN, p. 2, Aliso Vieho, CA: Author.

American Nurses Association (1980). *The nursing practice act: Suggested state legislation.* Kansas City, MO: Author.

American Nurses Association (1985). *Code of ethics for nurses with interpretive statements.* Kansas City, MO: Author.

American Nurses Association (1991). *Position statement on cultural diversity in nursing practice.* Kansas City, MO: Author.

American Nurses Association (1991). *Position statement on ethics and human rights.* Kansas City, MO: Author.

American Nurses Association (1991). *Standards of clinical practice.* Kansas City, MO: Author.

American Nurses Association (1993) Position statement on registered nurse utilization of assistive personnel. *American Nurse, 25*(2), 7–8.

American Nurses Association (1994). *Registered professional nurses and unlicensed assistive personnel.* Washington, DC: Author.

American Nurses Association (1995). *Nursing: A social policy statement.* Kansas City, MO: Author

Barrett, M. (1992). Optimizing nursing information systems. *Journal of Nursing Administration, 22*(10):60–67.

Bates, B. (1995). *A guide to physical examination* (6th ed.). Philadelphia: J.B. Lippincott.

Benner, P. (1984). *From novice to expert.* Menlo Park, CA: Addison-Wesley Publishers.

Berry, R. (1993). Effective patient education, part 1: Teaching adults. *Nursing Spectrum* (PA Ed), *2*(23),14–16.

Berry, R. (1993). Effective patient education, part 2: Teaching children. *Nursing Spectrum* (PA Ed), *2*(24), 14–15.

Birdshall, C., and Sperry, S. (1997). *Clinical paths in medical-surgical practice.* St. Louis: Mosby–Year Book.

Brigham, C. (1993). Nursing education and critical thinking: Interplay of content and thinking. *Holistic Health Nurse Practice, 7*(3), 48–54.

Brookfield, S. (1987) *Developing critical thinkers.* San Francisco: Jossey-Bass.

Bulechek, G., & McClosky, J. (1992). *Nursing interventions* (2nd ed.). Philadelphia: W.B. Saunders.

Burfitt, S., Greiner, D., & Miers, L. (1993). Professional nurse caring as perceived by critically ill patients: A phenomenologic study. *American Journal of Critical Care, 2*(6), 489–549

Burke, L., & Murphy, J. (1988). *Charting by exception: A cost-effective, quality approach.* Albany, NY: Delmar.

Campinha-Bacote, J. The quest for cultural competence in nursing care. *Nursing Forum, 30*(4):19–25.

Canadian Nurses Association (1987). *A definition of nursing practice: Standards for nursing practice.* Publication No. ISBNB 0-919 108-52-2. Ottawa, Canada: Author.

Carpenito, L. (1997a). *Handbook of nursing diagnosis* (7th ed.). Philadelphia: Lippincott-Raven.

Carpenito, L. (1997b). *Nursing diagnosis: Application to clinical practice* (7th ed.). Philadelphia: Lippincott-Raven.

Community Health Accreditation Program (CHAP). (1993). *Standards for excellence for home care organizations.* #21-2327, New York: National League for Nurses and CHAP.

Clark, A., & Garry, M., (1991). Legal implications of standards of care. *Dimensions of Critical Care Nursing, 10*(2), 96–102.

Covey, S. (1989). *The seven habits of highly effective people.* New York: Simon & Schuster.

Craft-Rosenberg, M., & Delaney, C. (1997). The keystone to a unified language. In M. Rentz & P. LeMone (eds.). *Classification of nursing diagnosis: Proceedings of the Twelfth National Conference*. Glendale, CA: CINAHL.

Fields, S. (1991). History-taking in the elderly: Obtaining useful information. *Geriatrics, 46*(8), 26–34.

Fitzpatrick, J. (1991). The translation of the NANDA taxonomy into ICD code. In R. M. Carroll-Johnson (Ed.). *Classification of nursing diagnoses: Proceedings of the Ninth National Conference* (pp. 19–22). Philadelphia: J.B. Lippincott.

Foster, P. (1993). Helping students learn to make ethical decisions. *Holistic Nurse Practice, 7*(3), 28–35.

Gebbie, K. (1975). *Classification of nursing diagnoses: Proceedings of the Second National Conference*. St. Louis, MO: National Clearinghouse for Nursing Diagnosis.

Gebbie, K., & Lavin, M. (Eds.). (1975). *Classification of nursing diagnoses: Proceedings of the First National Conference*. St. Louis, MO: C.V. Mosby–Year Book.

Gordon, M. (1994). *Nursing diagnosis: Process and application* (3rd ed.). St. Louis, MO: Mosby–Year Book.

Gray, B. (1995). What heals? *Critical Care Nurse* (Supplement). June 1995. 3–16.

Gryfinski, J., & Lampe, S. (1990). Implementing focus charting: Process and critique. *Clinical Nurse Specialist, 4*(4), 201–205.

Halpern, D. (1984). *Thought and knowledge: An introduction to critical thinking*. Hilldale, NJ: Lawrence Erlbaum Associates.

Hansen, R., & Washburn, M. (1995). Knowing how to delegate. *American Journal of Nursing, 95*(7), 16H–16I.

Henderson, V. (1961). *Basic principles of nursing care*. London: International Council of Nurses.

Hoffman, L., Wesmiller, S., Sciurba, F., Johnson, J., Ferson, P., Zullo, T., & Dauber, M. (1992). Nasal cannula and transtracheal oxygen delivery: A comparison of patient response after 6 months of each technique. *American Review of Respiratory Disease, 145*(4), 827–831.

Iowa Intervention Project—McCloskey, J., & Bulechek, G. M. (Eds.). (1996). *Nursing interventions classification (NIC)* (2nd ed.). St. Louis, MO: Mosby–Year Book.

Iyer, P., & Camp, N. (1995). *Nursing documentation: A nursing process approach* (2nd ed.). St. Louis, MO: C.V. Mosby–Year Book.

Jackson, L. (1993). Understanding, eliciting and negotiating clients' multicultural health beliefs. *Nurse Practitioner American Journal of Primary Health Care, 18*(4), 30, 32, 37–38.

Johnson, M., & Maas, M. Nursing-sensitive outcomes classification: An overview. (1997). In M. Rentz & P. LeMone. (eds.) *Classification of nursing diagnosis: Proceedings of the Twelfth National Conference*. Glendale, CA: CINAHL.

Johnson, S., Scott, M., & Quinn, S. (1995). New graduates transitioning into home care. *Nursing Spectrum, 4*(24), 7.

Joint Commission on Accreditation of Healthcare Organizations (1992). *1993 Accreditation manual for hospitals*. Oakbrook Terrace, IL: Author.

Joint Commission on Accreditation of Healthcare Organizations (1994). *Accreditation manual for hospitals*. Oakbrook Terrace, IL: Author.

Jones, J. A. (1988). Clinical reasoning: Ethics, science, art. *Journal of Advanced Nursing, 13*(2), 185–192.

Kahnl, K., Ivaninc, L., & Fuhrmann, M. (1992). Automated nursing documentation system provides a favorable return on investment. *Journal of Nursing Administration, 21*(11), 44–51.

Krumberger, J. (1996). Culture—An inextricable component of care. *Critical Care Nurse, 16*(3), 118.

Lampe, S. (1990). Focus charting: Streamlining documentation. *Nursing Management, 16*(7), 44.

Leininger, M. (1994). Quality of life from a transcultural nursing perspective. *Nursing Science Quarterly, 7*(1), 22–28.SS

Maslow, A. (1970). *Motivation in personality*. New York: Harper & Row.

Milstead, J., & Rodrigues-Fisher, L. (1992). Legally defensible, effective charting. *Critical Care Nurse, 12*(6), 103–105.

North American Nursing Diagnosis Association. (1994). *Nursing diagnoses: Definitions and classification 1995–1996*. Philadelphia: Author.

Orem, D. (1980). *Nursing: Concepts of practice* (2nd ed.). New York: McGraw-Hill.

Parkman, C. (1996). Delegation. *American Journal of Nursing, 96*(9), 43–47.

Paul, R., & Binker, A. (Eds.). (1990). *Critical thinking: What every person needs to survive in a rapidly changing world*. Rohner Park, CA: Foundation for Critical thinking and Moral Development.

Rehabilitation Nursing Foundation's Nursing Diagnosis Publications Task Force (1995). *21 Rehabilitation Nursing Diagnoses*. Glenview, IL: Rehabilitation Nursing Foundation.

Rentz, M., & LeMone, P. (1997). *Classification of nursing diagnosis: Proceedings of the Twelfth National Conference*. Glendale, CA: CINAHL.

Ruggiero, V. (1991). *The art of thinking: A guide to critical and creative thought* (3rd ed.). New York: Harper Collins.

Secretary's Commission on Achieving Necessary Skills. (1992). *Learning a Living: A blueprint for high performance, a SCANS report for America 2000.* The U.S. Department of Labor,

Taylor, C., Lillis, C., & LeMone, P. (1997). *Fundamentals of nursing: The art and science of nursing care* (3rd ed.). Philadelphia: J.B. Lippincott.

U.S. Department of Health and Human Services, Public Health Service (1990). *Healthy people 2000.* DHHS Publication No. (PHS) 91-50212. Washington, DC: Superintendent of Documents, U.S. Government Printing Office.

Wells, S. (1996). Adding an "at home" path to your discharge plan. *American Journal of Nursing, 96*(10), 73–74.

Wilkinson, J. (1996). *Nursing process: A critical thinking approach* (2nd ed.). Menlo Park, CA: Addison-Wesley.

Zander, K. (1988), Nursing case management: Strategic management of cost and quality outcomes. *Journal of Nursing Administration, 18*(5), 32–38.

Ziegler, S., Vaughan-Wroble, B., & Erlen, J. (1986). *Nursing process, nursing knowledge: Avenues to autonomy.* Norwalk, CT: Appleton & Lange.

Zimmerman, P. (1996). Delegating to unlicensed assistive personnel. *Nursing Spectrum* (FL Ed), *6*(12): 12–13.

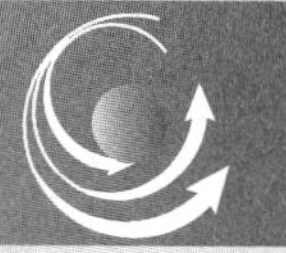

QUICK REFERENCE TO

Nursing Diagnoses

Organized alphabetically, this section is designed to provide you with easy access to basic information about each of the diagnoses accepted for clinical testing by the North American Nursing Diagnosis Association (NANDA). The definitions are NANDA definitions unless otherwise stated, with minor adaptation in some cases for clarity. The information listed under the heading *Related Factors* and *Defining Characteristics* has been adapted from NANDA *Nursing Diagnosis: Definitions and Classifications 1995–1996*. New diagnoses listed as of 1997 are also included, as well as two diagnoses that have been added by myself (*Grieving* and *Impaired Communication*).

Alphabetical Listing of Diagnoses Accepted for Testing by NANDA

Activity Intolerance
Activity Intolerance, Risk for
Adaptive Capacity: Intracranial, Decreased
Adjustment, Impaired
Airway Clearance, Ineffective
Anxiety
Aspiration, Risk for

Body Image Disturbance
Body Temperature, Risk for Altered
Bowel Incontinence
Breastfeeding, Effective
Breastfeeding, Ineffective
Breastfeeding, Interrupted
Breathing Pattern, Ineffective

Cardiac Output, Decreased
Caregiver Role Strain
Caregiver Role Strain, Risk for
Communication, Impaired*
Communication, Impaired Verbal
Community Coping, Ineffective
Community Coping, Potential for Enhanced
Confusion, Acute
Confusion, Chronic
Constipation
Constipation, Colonic
Constipation, Perceived
Coping, Defensive
Coping, Ineffective Individual

Decisional Conflict (Specify)
Denial, Ineffective
Diarrhea
Disuse Syndrome, Risk for
Diversional Activity Deficit
Dysreflexia

Energy Field Disturbance
Environmental Interpretation Syndrome, Impaired

Family Coping: Compromised, Ineffective
Family Coping: Disabling, Ineffective
Family Coping: Potential for Growth
Family Process: Alcoholism, Altered
Family Processes, Altered
Fatigue
Fear

*Not on the list as of 1997; added by author.

Fluid Volume Deficit
Fluid Volume Deficit, Risk for
Fluid Volume Excess

Gas Exchange, Impaired
Grieving*
Grieving, Anticipatory
Grieving, Dysfunctional
Growth and Development, Altered

Health Seeking Behaviors (Specify)
Health Maintenance, Altered
Home Maintenance Management, Impaired
Hopelessness
Hyperthermia
Hypothermia

Infant Behavior, Disorganized
Infant Behavior, Disorganized, Risk for
Infant Behavior, Potential for Enhanced Organized
Infant Feeding Pattern, Ineffective
Infection, Risk for
Injury, Risk for

Knowledge Deficit (Specify)

Loneliness, Risk for

Mobility, Impaired Physical

Noncompliance (Specify)
Memory, Impaired
Nutrition, Altered: Less than Body Requirements
Nutrition, Altered: More than Body Requirements
Nutrition, Altered: Risk for More than Body Requirements

Oral Mucous Membrane, Altered

Pain
Pain, Chronic
Parental Role Conflict
Parent/Infant/Child Attachment, Risk for Altered
Parenting, Altered
Parenting, Risk for Altered
Perioperative Positioning Injury, Risk for
Peripheral Neurovascular Dysfunction, Risk for
Personal Identity Disturbance

*Not on the list as of 1997; added by author.

Poisoning, Risk for
Post-Trauma Response
Powerlessness
Protection, Altered

Rape-Trauma Syndrome†
Relocation Stress Syndrome
Role Performance, Altered

Self Care Deficit, Bathing/Hygiene
Self Care Deficit, Dressing/Grooming
Self Care Deficit, Feeding
Self Care Deficit, Toileting
Self Esteem, Chronic Low
Self Esteem, Disturbance
Self Esteem, Situational Low
Self-Mutilation, Risk for
Sensory/Perceptual Alterations (Specify: visual, auditory, kinesthetic, gustatory, tactile, olfactory)
Sexual Dysfunction
Sexuality Patterns, Altered
Skin Integrity, Impaired
Skin Integrity, Risk for Impaired
Sleep Pattern Disturbance
Social Interaction, Impaired
Social Isolation
Spiritual Distress
Spiritual Well-Being, Potential for Enhanced
Suffocation, Risk for
Swallowing, Impaired

Therapeutic Regimen: Community, Ineffective Management of
Therapeutic Regimen: Families, Ineffective Management of
Therapeutic Regimen: Individual, Effective Management of
Therapeutic Regimen: Individual, Ineffective Management of
Thermoregulation, Ineffective
Thought Processes, Altered
Tissue Integrity, Impaired
Tissue Perfusion, Altered (Specify: renal, cerebral, cardiopulmonary, gastrointestinal, peripheral)
Trauma, Risk for

† NANDA has this listed as three different diagnoses (*Rape Trauma Syndrome, Rape Trauma Syndrome: Silent Reaction, Rape Trauma Syndrome: Compound Reaction*), all with the same definition.

Unilateral Neglect
Urinary Elimination, Altered
Urinary Incontinence, Functional
Urinary Incontinence, Reflex
Urinary Incontinence, Stress
Urinary Incontinence, Total
Urinary Incontinence, Urge
Urinary Retention

Ventilation, Inability to Sustain Spontaneous
Ventilatory Weaning Response, Dysfunctional (DVWR)
Violence, Risk for: Self-directed or Directed at Others

Activity Intolerance

A state in which an individual has insufficient energy to endure or complete required or desired daily activities.

• Related Factors

Deconditioned state (bed rest or immobility), generalized weakness, sedentary lifestyle, aging process, disease process (imbalance between oxygen supply and demand, acute or chronic illness), medication side effects.

• Defining Characteristics

— *SUBJECTIVE DATA* (reported) —

Weakness or fatigue, exertional discomfort or dyspnea, reduced ability to perform desired activities.

— *OBJECTIVE DATA* (observed) —

Abnormal heart rate and blood pressure response to activity, electrocardiograph changes reflecting arrhythmias or ischemia.

• Clinical Alert

Activity Intolerance is often related to compromised respiratory, cardiac, or circulatory function.

• Compare With

Activity Intolerance, Risk for; Disuse Syndrome, Risk for; Fatigue.

Activity Intolerance, Risk for

A state in which an individual is at risk for experiencing insufficient energy to endure or complete required or desired daily activities.

• Risk Factors

See related factors for *Activity Intolerance*.

Adaptive Capacity: Intracranial, Decreased

The state in which a person's intracranial fluid dynamic mechanisms that normally compensate for increases in intracranial volumes are compromised, resulting in repeated disproportionate increases in intracranial pressure (ICP) in response to a variety of noxious and non-noxious stimuli.

• Related Factors

Brain injuries, sustained increase in ICP ≥10–15 mmHg, decreased cerebral perfusion pressure ≤50–60 mmHg, systemic hypotension with intracranial hypertension.

• Defining Characteristics

— *OBJECTIVE DATA* (observed) —

Repeated increases in ICP >10 mmHg for more than 5 minutes following a variety of external stimuli, disproportionate increase in ICP following single environmental or nursing maneuver stimulus, elevated P2 ICP waveform, volume pressure response test variation (Volume-pressure ratio >2, pressure=volume index <10), baseline ICP ≥10 mmHg, wide amplitude ICP waveform.

Adjustment, Impaired

The state in which a person is unable to modify his or her lifestyle or behavior in a manner that promotes adaptation to a change in health status.

• Related Factors

Disability requiring change in lifestyle, inadequate support systems, impaired cognition, sensory overload, assault to self-esteem, altered locus of control, incomplete grieving.

• Defining Characteristics

— *SUBJECTIVE DATA* (reported) —

Nonacceptance of health status change; extended period of shock, disbelief, or anger regarding health status change; lack of future-oriented thinking.

— *OBJECTIVE DATA* (observed) —

Nonexistent or ineffective involvement in problem solving or goal setting, lack of movement toward independence.

• Compare With

Coping, Ineffective Individual; Grieving, Dysfunctional; Self-Esteem Disturbance.

Airway Clearance, Ineffective

A state in which a person is unable to clear secretions or obstructions from the respiratory tract to maintain airway patency.

• Related Factors

Neuromuscular impairment; respiratory infections; upper airway obstruction; excessive secretions; thick secretions; sedation; decreased energy or fatigue; chest pain, incisional pain; perceptual or cognitive impairment; *Knowledge Deficit (effective coughing techniques).*

• Defining Characteristics

— *SUBJECTIVE DATA* (reported) —

Dyspnea, report of inability to cough up secretions, fear of coughing, pain with coughing.

— *OBJECTIVE DATA* (observed) —

Cough that doesn't clear airway; abnormal breath sounds; abnormal rate, rhythm, or depth of respirations; tachypnea; tachycardia; decreased oxygen saturation level.

• Compare With

Aspiration, Risk for; Breathing Pattern, Ineffective.

Anxiety

The state in which a person experiences an uneasiness (mild or intense), the source of which is often nonspecific or unknown to the individual.

• Related Factors

Conscious or unconscious conflict about essential values or life goals; actual or perceived threat to self-concept, role function, security, or usual interaction patterns; situational or maturational crisis (eg, pregnancy, parenting); multiple stressors or demands; sleep deprivation; fear of pain, loneliness, physical or psychological harm; inability to cope with or control situations; loss(es).

• Defining Characteristics

— *SUBJECTIVE DATA* (reported) —

Nervousness, tension; inability to relax, concentrate, or make decisions; lack of self-confidence; feelings of uncertainty, helplessness, or inadequacy; insomnia; somatic discomfort (eg, diarrhea, headache, chest discomfort); changes in eating habits.

— *OBJECTIVE DATA* (observed) —

Restlessness; increased perspiration, pulse rate, and blood pressure; pallor; tremors; extraneous movements, lack of initiative, self-deprecation, poor eye contact.

• Clinical Alert

Sudden onset of anxiety, especially in the elderly, may be an early symptom of hypotension, hypoxemia, sepsis, or coronary disorders. Monitor vital signs carefully.

• Compare With

Fear.

Aspiration, Risk for

The state in which a person is at risk for entry of gastrointestinal (GI) or oropharyngeal secretions, or solids or fluids into the tracheobronchial passages.

• Risk Factors

Reduced level of consciousness; depressed cough and gag reflexes; impaired swallowing; presence of tracheostomy or endotracheal tube; incompetent lower esophageal sphincter; increased intragastric pressure; increased gastric residual; decreased GI motility; delayed gastric emptying; GI immaturity (infants); GI tubes; tube feedings; medication administration; situations hindering elevation of upper body; facial, oral, or neck surgery or trauma; wired jaws.

• Compare With

Airway Clearance, Ineffective; Suffocation, Risk for; Swallowing, Impaired.

Body Image Disturbance

The state in which a person experiences a disruption in perception of body image.

• Related Factors

Biophysical factors, such as pregnancy, chronic disease, obesity, body changes related to adolescence or aging, loss of body part or function, effects of radiation or chemotherapy; cognitive or perceptual factors, such as inaccurate interpretation of body or body parts; psychosocial, cultural, or spiritual factors.

• Defining Characteristics

— ***SUBJECTIVE DATA*** (reported) —

Unwanted change in appearance or lifestyle; fear of rejection or reaction by others, or negative feelings about body; focus on past strength, function, or appearance; emphasis on remaining strengths, heightened achievement; preoccupation with change or loss; expansion of body boundary to incorporate environmental objects; personalization of part or loss by name; depersonalization of part or loss by impersonal pronouns; refusal to verify actual change.

— ***OBJECTIVE DATA*** (observed) —

Missing body part, change in structure or function, not looking at body part, not touching body part, hiding or overexposing body part (intentional or unintentional), trauma to nonfunctioning part, change in social involvement, change in ability to estimate spatial relationship of body to environment.

• Compare With

Self-Esteem Disturbance.

Body Temperature, Risk for Altered

The state in which a person is at risk for failure to maintain body temperature within normal range.

• Risk Factors

Extremes of age, extremes of weight, exposure to cold or hot environments, dehydration, inactivity or vigorous activity, medications causing vasoconstriction or vasodilation, altered metabolic rate, sedation, inappropriate clothing for environmental temperature, illness or trauma affecting temperature regulation, infection.

• Compare With

Hyperthermia; Hypothermia; Thermoregulation, Ineffective.

Bowel Incontinence

A state in which a person experiences a change in normal bowel habits characterized by involuntary passage of stool.

• Related Factors

Loss of sphincter control, neuromuscular disorder, inflammatory bowel disease, decreased level of consciousness, confusion, progressive dementia, depression, *Anxiety, Diarrhea.*

• Defining Characteristics

— ***OBJECTIVE DATA*** (observed) —

Involuntary passage of stool.

• Compare With

Diarrhea.

Breastfeeding, Effective

The state in which a mother–infant dyad exhibits adequate proficiency and satisfaction with the breastfeeding process.

• Related Factors

Mother: basic breastfeeding knowledge, normal breast structure, maternal confidence.
Infant: gestational age greater than 34 weeks, normal oral structure.

• Defining Characteristics

— ***SUBJECTIVE DATA*** (reported) —

Satisfaction with the breastfeeding process.

— ***OBJECTIVE DATA*** (observed) —

Mother: able to position infant at breast to promote a successful latch-on response, signs of oxytocin release (ie, let-down, or milk ejection, reflex), effective mother–infant communication patterns (ie, infant cues, mother interprets and responds).
Infant: contentment after feeding, regular and sustained suckling and swallowing at the breast, appropriate weight gain for age, adequate elimination patterns for age, eagerness to nurse.

• Compare With

Breastfeeding, Ineffective; Breastfeeding, Interrupted.

Breastfeeding, Ineffective

The state in which a mother and infant or child experience dissatisfaction or difficulty with the breastfeeding process.

• Related Factors

Mother: frequent supplemental feedings with artificial nipple, lack of basic breastfeeding knowledge, history of breastfeeding difficulty or failure, interrupted breastfeeding, previous breast surgery, inverted or painful nipples, engorged breasts, maternal diet inadequate in nutrients or fluids, nonsupportive partner or family, maternal anxiety or ambivalence.
Infant: gestational age less than 34 weeks, structural anomaly, poor sucking reflex.

• Defining Characteristics

— *SUBJECTIVE DATA* (reported) —

Unsatisfactory breastfeeding process, inadequate milk supply, persistence of sore nipples beyond first week of breastfeeding.

— *OBJECTIVE DATA* (observed) —

Mother: insufficient emptying of breast, no observable signs of oxytocin release (ie, let-down, or milk ejection, reflex), inadequate milk supply.
Infant: inability to latch onto breast; arching and crying at the breast; nonsustained suckling; insufficient opportunity for suckling; fussing, crying, and unresponsiveness to comfort measures within the first hour after feeding; weight loss, or failure to gain.

• Compare With

Breastfeeding, Effective; Breastfeeding, Interrupted; Infant Feeding Pattern, Ineffective.

Breastfeeding, Interrupted

A break in the continuity of the breastfeeding process as a result of inability or inadvisability to put baby to breast for feeding.

• Related Factors

Maternal or infant illness, prematurity, maternal employment, contraindication to breastfeeding (eg, drugs, true breast milk jaundice), need to abruptly wean infant.

• Defining Characteristics

— *SUBJECTIVE DATA* (reported) —

Desire to maintain lactation and provide (or eventually provide) breast milk for infant's nutritional needs.

— *OBJECTIVE DATA* (observed) —

Infant doesn't receive milk from breast for some or all of feedings, mother–infant separation, lack of knowledge regarding expression and storage of breast milk.

• Compare With

Breastfeeding, Effective; Breastfeeding, Ineffective; Infant Feeding Pattern, Ineffective.

Breathing Pattern, Ineffective

The state in which a person's inhalation or exhalation pattern does not promote adequate ventilation.

• Related Factors

Neuromuscular impairment, obstructive lung disease, restrictive lung disease, musculoskeletal impairment, decreased energy, *Fatigue, Anxiety, Pain,* medication side effects (respiratory depression).

• Defining Characteristics

— *SUBJECTIVE DATA* (reported) —

Dyspnea, shortness of breath.

— *OBJECTIVE DATA* (observed) —

Changes in respiratory rate or depth of respirations; changes in pulse rate or rhythm; wheezing; fremitus; cough; nasal flaring; cyanosis; decreased diaphragmatic excursion; assumption of three-point position; use of accessory muscles; orthopnea; abnormal arterial blood gases; reduced vital capacity, forced-end expiratory volume, or oxygen saturation level; splinted or guarded respirations.

• Clinical Alert

Report persistent *Ineffective Breathing Pattern* not responding to nurse-prescribed interventions immediately. This is especially important if confusion or severe anxiety is present, because both of these are signs of hypoxemia.

• Compare With

Activity Intolerance; Airway Clearance, Ineffective.

Cardiac Output, Decreased

A state in which a person's heart is unable to pump blood with enough force to meet the needs of the body's tissues.

• Related Factors

Dehydration, cardiac pathology (eg, left ventricular failure), medication side effects.

• Defining Characteristics

— *SUBJECTIVE DATA* (reported) —

Fatigue, vertigo, dyspnea, orthopnea.

— *OBJECTIVE DATA* (observed) —

Low blood pressure; rapid heart rate; arrhythmias; angina; jugular vein distention; cyanosis of skin and mucous membranes; dependent edema; oliguria; decreased peripheral pulses; cold, clammy skin; rales; restlessness.

• Author's Note

The defining characteristics of this problem represent a *collaborative problem,* rather than a *nursing diagnosis.*

• Compare With

Activity Intolerance.

Caregiver Role Strain

The state in which a caregiver perceives difficulty in performing the family caregiver role.

• Related Factors

Care receiver: severity of or prolongation of illness, unpredictable illness course, early discharge from skilled nursing facility, complexity or amount of care needed.
Caregiver: lack of preparation or experience, impaired physical or mental health, lack of respite or recreation, competing role commitments.
Other Factors: inadequate physical environment, family dysfunction.

• Defining Characteristics

— *SUBJECTIVE DATA* (reported) —

Inadequate resources; difficulty performing caregiving activities; concern regarding outcome for the care receiver; conflict with other role responsibilities; family conflict around issues of providing care; feelings of stress, nervousness, and depression.

— *OBJECTIVE DATA* (observed) —

Reduction in quality of care, increased family discord, long hours of caregiving without time off.

Caregiver Role Strain, Risk for

The state in which a caregiver is at risk for perceiving difficulty in performing the family caregiver role.

• Risk Factors

See related factors for *Caregiver Role Strain.*

Communication, Impaired*

The state in which a person experiences a decreased ability to send or receive messages (ie, has difficulty exchanging thoughts, ideas, or desires) (Carpenito, 1997b, p. 227).

• Related Factors

Effects of cerebral impairment (expressive or receptive aphasia), hearing or auditory comprehension deficits, decreased ability to speak words, language barriers, lack of privacy, *Altered Thought Processes.*

• Defining Characteristics

— *SUBJECTIVE DATA* (reported) —

Concern about being able to make self understood, or to understand directions, reluctance to speak, difficulty understanding or speaking dominant language.

— *OBJECTIVE DATA* (observed) —

Repetition of questions without apparent understanding of answers; inappropriate (or absent) speech or response; incongruence between verbal and nonverbal messages; stuttering, slurring, word-finding problems; weak or absent voice; confusion; use of sign language.

---

*Not on the list as of 1997; added by author.

• Author's Note

Only *Impaired Verbal Communication* is on NANDA's list of diagnoses accepted for study. *Impaired Communication* has been included here because it includes a wider range of communication problems.

• Compare With

Communication, Impaired Verbal.

Communication, Impaired Verbal

The state in which a person experiences a decreased or absent ability to speak but can understand others (Carpenito, 1997b).

• Related Factors

Physical barrier (tracheostomy, intubation), anatomical defect (cleft lip or palate), brain injury or pathology causing expressive aphasia, psychological barriers (psychosis, fear), language barriers.

• Defining Characteristics

— *OBJECTIVE DATA* (observed) —

Difficulty with dominant language, speech, or verbalization; does not or cannot speak.

• Compare With

Communication, Impaired.

Community Coping, Ineffective

A pattern of community activities for adaptation and problem solving that is unsatisfactory for meeting the demands or needs of the community.

• Related Factors

Deficits in social support, inadequate resources for problem solving, powerlessness.

• Defining Characteristics

— *SUBJECTIVE DATA* (reported) —

Community does not meet its own expectations, expressed difficulty in meeting demands for change, expressed vulnerability, stressors perceived as excessive.

— *OBJECTIVE DATA* (observed) —

Deficits in community participation, deficits in communication methods, excessive community conflicts, high illness rates.

• Compare With

Community Coping, Potential for Enhanced; Therapeutic Regimen: Community, Ineffective Management of.

Community Coping, Potential for Enhanced

A pattern of community activities for adaptation and problem solving that is satisfactory for meeting the demands or needs of the community but can be improved for management of current and future problems/stressors.

• Related Factors

Social supports available, resources available for problem solving, community has a sense of power to manage stressors.

• Defining Characteristics

— *SUBJECTIVE DATA* (reported) —

Agreement that community is responsible for stress management.

— *OBJECTIVE DATA* (observed) —

Deficits in one or more characteristics that indicate effective coping, active planning by community for predicted stressors, active problem solving by community when faced with issues, positive communication among community members, positive communication between community aggregates and larger community, programs available for recreation and relaxation, resources sufficient for managing stressors.

• Compare With

Community Coping, Ineffective; Therapeutic Regimen: Community, Ineffective Management of.

Confusion, Acute

The state in which a person experiences the abrupt onset of a cluster of global, transient changes and disturbances in attention, cognition, psychomotor activity, level of consciousness, and/or sleep–wake cycle.

• Related Factors

Age >60 years, dementia, alcohol abuse, drug abuse, delirium.

• Defining Characteristics

— *SUBJECTIVE DATA* (reported) —

Hallucinations.

— *OBJECTIVE DATA* (observed) —

Fluctuation in cognition, fluctuation in sleep–wake cycle, fluctuation in level of consciousness, fluctuation in psychomotor activity, increased agitation or restlessness, misperceptions, lack of motivation to initiate and/or follow through with goal-directed or purposeful behavior.

• Compare With

Confusion, Chronic; Environmental Interpretation Syndrome, Impaired; Sensory-Perceptual Alterations; Thought Processes, Altered.

Confusion, Chronic

The state in which a person experiences an irreversible, long-standing, and/or progressive deterioration of intellect and personality characterized by decreased ability to interpret environmental stimuli, decreased capacity for intellectual thought processes and manifested by disturbances of memory, orientation, and behavior.

• Related Factors

Alzheimer's disease, Korsakoff's psychosis, multi-infarct dementia, cerebral vascular accident, head injury.

• Defining Characteristics

— *OBJECTIVE DATA* (observed) —

Clinical evidence of organic impairment, altered interpretation/response to stimuli, progressive/long-standing cognitive impairment, no change in level of consciousness, impaired socialization, impaired memory (short term, long term), altered personality.

• Compare With

Confusion, Acute; Environmental Interpretation Syndrome, Impaired; Sensory-Perceptual Alterations; Thought Processes, Altered.

Constipation

A state in which a person experiences a change in normal bowel habits characterized by a decrease in frequency of defecation or passage of hard, dry stools.

• Related Factors

Bed rest, diet deficient in fluids or roughage, lack of exercise, lack of privacy, laxative dependence, painful defecation, pregnancy, side effects of medications, neuromuscular impairment.

• Defining Characteristics

— *SUBJECTIVE DATA* (reported) —

Feeling of rectal pressure or fullness, headache, abdominal pain, back pain, decreased appetite, nausea.

— *OBJECTIVE DATA* (observed) —

Decreased frequency of stools; hard, formed stools; straining at stool; palpable rectal mass.

• Clinical Alert

Untreated constipation can lead to fecal impaction and intestinal obstruction.

• Compare With

Constipation, Perceived; Constipation, Colonic.

Constipation, Colonic

The state in which a person's pattern of elimination is characterized by hard, dry stool that results from a delay in passage of food residue.

• Related Factors

Less than adequate fluid intake, less than adequate dietary intake, less than adequate fiber, less than adequate physical activity, immobility, lack of privacy, emotional disturbances, chronic use of laxatives and enemas, stress, change in daily routine.

• Defining Characteristics

— *SUBJECTIVE DATA* (reported) —

Painful defecation, abdominal pain, rectal pressure, headache, decreased appetite.

— *OBJECTIVE DATA* (observed) —

Decreased frequency of stools; hard, dry stools; straining at stool; abdominal distention; palpable rectal mass.

• Compare With

Constipation; Constipation, Perceived.

Constipation, Perceived

The state in which a person makes a self-diagnosis of constipation when constipation does not exist, and ensures a daily bowel movement through abuse of laxatives, enemas, and suppositories.

• Related Factors

Cultural or family health beliefs, faulty appraisal, impaired thought processes, obsessive–compulsive disorders.

• Defining Characteristics

— *SUBJECTIVE DATA* (reported) —

Expectation of a daily bowel movement with the resulting overuse of laxatives, enemas, and suppositories; expected passage of stool at same time every day.

• Compare With

Constipation; Constipation, Colonic.

Coping, Defensive

The state in which a person repeatedly projects falsely positive self-evaluation based on a self-protective pattern that defends against underlying perceived threats to positive self-regard.

• Related Factors

Loss of job or ability to work, financial problems, marital problems, failure in school, legal problems, institutionalization, *Fear,* aging.

• Defining Characteristics

— *OBJECTIVE DATA* (observed) —

Denial of obvious problems or weaknesses, rationalization, hypersensitivity to criticism, grandiosity, projection of blame or responsibility, superior attitude toward others, difficulty establishing or maintaining relationships, hostile laughter or ridicule of others, difficulty in reality testing perceptions, lack of follow-through or participation in treatment or therapy.

• Compare With

Coping, Ineffective Individual; Self-Esteem Disturbance.

Coping, Ineffective Individual

The state in which a person experiences impaired adaptive behaviors and problem-solving abilities in meeting demands and roles of life.

• Related Factors

Situational or maturational crises, persistent stress, sensory overload, personal vulnerability, poor self-esteem, inadequate or unavailable support system, conflict with values or beliefs.

• Defining Characteristics

— *SUBJECTIVE DATA* (reported) —

Inability to cope or inability to ask for help.

— *OBJECTIVE DATA* (observed) —

Inability to meet role expectations or solve problems, altered societal participation, destructive behavior toward self or others, inappropriate use of defense mechanism, change in usual communication patterns, manipulative behavior, high illness or accident rate.

• Compare With

Adjustment, Impaired; Coping, Defensive; Denial, Ineffective.

Decisional Conflict (Specify)

The state in which a person experiences uncertainty about the course of action to be taken when choices involve risk, loss, or challenge to personal life values.

• Related Factors

Unclear personal values or beliefs, perceived threat to value system, lack of experience or interference with decision making, lack of relevant information, support system deficit, multiple or divergent sources of information.

• Defining Characteristics

— *SUBJECTIVE DATA* (reported) —

Uncertainty about choices, concern about undesired consequences of actions being considered, vacillation between choices, delayed decision making, feeling of distress while attempting a decision, self-focusing, questioning of personal values and beliefs while attempting a decision.

— *OBJECTIVE DATA* (observed) —

Signs of distress or tension (eg, increased heart rate, increased muscle tension, restlessness, and so forth).

• Compare With

Coping, Ineffective Individual; Spiritual Distress.

Denial, Ineffective

The state of a conscious or unconscious attempt to disavow the knowledge or meaning of an event to reduce anxiety or fear to the detriment of health.

• Related Factors

Illness or addiction accompanied by fear of death, separation, or loss of autonomy; *Anxiety.*

• Defining Characteristics

— *SUBJECTIVE DATA* (reported) —

Failure to perceive personal relevance of symptoms or danger, minimizing of symptoms, displacement of symptoms to other organs, displacement of fear or impact of the condition, inability to admit impact of disease on life pattern.

— *OBJECTIVE DATA* (observed) —

Lack of verbalization of fear of death or invalidism, delay in seeking (or refusal to accept) health care to the detriment of health, use of home remedies or self-medication to relieve symptoms, use of dismissive gestures or comments when speaking of distressing events, inappropriate affect.

• Compare With

Adjustment, Impaired; Coping, Defensive; Coping, Ineffective Individual.

Diarrhea

A state in which a person experiences a change in normal bowel habits characterized by the frequent passage of loose, fluid, unformed stools.

• Related Factors

Side effects of medications or radiation therapy, tube feedings, inflammatory or malabsorptive disorders, infectious processes, food intolerances, *Anxiety.*

• Defining Characteristics

— *SUBJECTIVE DATA* (reported) —

Abdominal pain, cramping, urgency.

— *OBJECTIVE DATA* (observed) —

Loose liquid stools, increased frequency of stools, increased frequency of bowel sounds.

• Compare With

Bowel Incontinence.

Disuse Syndrome, Risk for

A state in which a person is at risk for deterioration of body systems as the result of musculoskeletal inactivity.

• Risk Factors

Neuromuscular impairment (eg, paralysis, multiple sclerosis), musculoskeletal disorders, mechanical immobilization, prescribed immobilization, severe pain, altered level of consciousness, psychiatric disorders.

• Author's Note

This diagnosis is appropriate when interventions are aimed at promoting physiologic and psychosocial integrity, and preventing complications of immobility.

• Compare With

Mobility, Impaired Physical.

Diversional Activity Deficit

The state in which a person experiences a decreased stimulation from (or interest or engagement in) recreational or leisure activities.

• Related Factors

Lack of diversional activity (eg, long-term hospitalization, frequent lengthy treatments), sight or hearing loss, inability to participate in usual activities, retirement.

• Defining Characteristics

— *SUBJECTIVE DATA* (reported) —

Boredom or disinterest.

— *OBJECTIVE DATA* (observed) —

Flat affect, restlessness, hostility.

Dysreflexia

The state in which a person with a spinal cord injury at T7 or above experiences a life-threatening, uninhibited, sympathetic response of the nervous system to a noxious stimulus.

• Related Factors

Bladder or bowel distention (nonpatent catheter, bladder infection, constipation, impaction); spastic sphincter; acute abdomen, abdominal or thigh skin stimulation; lack of knowledge of prevention.

• Defining Characteristics

— *SUBJECTIVE DATA* (reported) —

Headache (a diffuse pain in different portions of the head and not confined to any nerve distribution area), chilling, paresthesia, blurred vision, chest pain, metallic taste, nasal congestion.

— *OBJECTIVE DATA* (observed) —

Individual with spinal cord injury at T7 or above with: paroxysmal hypertension (sudden periodic elevated blood pressure, systolic pressure over 140 mmHg and diastolic above 90 mmHg); bradycardia or tachycardia (pulse rate of less than 60 or over 100 beats per minute); diaphoresis or red splotches on skin (above the injury); pallor (below the injury); conjunctival congestion; Horner syndrome (contraction of the pupil, partial ptosis of the eyelid, enophthalmos and sometimes loss of sweating over the affected side of the face); pilomotor reflex (gooseflesh formation when skin is cooled).

• Clinical Alert

This diagnosis is most useful as a *risk diagnosis.* If *actual* dysreflexia is noted, immediate corrective measures must be initiated (eg, raising the head of the bed, removing or correcting factors listed under related factors). If the condition doesn't respond promptly to initial treatment, emergency treatment with pharmacologic intervention is likely to be required.

Energy Field Disturbance

A state in which the flow of energy surrounding a person's being is disrupted, resulting in a disharmony of the body, mind, and/or spirit.

• Related Factors

(None listed.)

• Defining Characteristics

— *SUBJECTIVE DATA* (reported) —

Temperature change (warmth/coolness), visual changes (image/color), disruption of the field (vacant/hold/spike/bulge), movement (wave/spike/tingling/dense/flowing), sounds (tone/words).

Environmental Interpretation Syndrome, Impaired

The state in which a person experiences a consistent lack of orientation to person, place, time, or circumstances for more than 3 to 6 months, necessitating a protective environment.

• Related Factors

Dementia (Alzheimer's disease, multi-infarct dementia, Pick's disease, AIDS dementia), Parkinson's disease, Huntington's disease, depression, alcoholism.

• Defining Characteristics

— *OBJECTIVE DATA* (observed) —

Consistent disorientation in known and unknown environments, chronic confusional states, loss of occupation or social functioning from memory decline, inability to follow simple directions or instructions, inability to reason or concentrate, slow response to questions.

• Compare With

Confusion, Acute; Confusion, Chronic; Sensory-Perceptual Alteration; Thought Processes, Altered.

Family Coping: Compromised, Ineffective

The state in which usually supportive significant others provide insufficient, ineffective, or compromised support, comfort, assistance, or encouragement to someone with a health challenge.

• Related Factors

Inadequate or incorrect information or understanding by a primary support person, preoccupation with emotional conflicts and personal suffering, temporary family disorganization and role changes, concurrent situations or crises, inability of significant others to provide support with health challenge, prolonged disease or disability.

• Defining Characteristics

— *SUBJECTIVE DATA* (reported) —

Concern about response of significant other(s), significant other(s) describes preoccupation with personal reaction or inadequate knowledge or understanding of health challenge.

— *OBJECTIVE DATA* (observed) —

Withdrawal or limited contact by significant other(s), inappropriate assistance or supportive behaviors, unrealistic expectations for abilities of challenged individual, overprotection of challenged individual.

• Compare With

Family Coping: Disabling, Ineffective; Family Processes, Altered; Parental Role Conflict; Parenting, Altered.

Family Coping: Disabling, Ineffective

The state in which a family demonstrates destructive behavior in response to an inability to manage internal or external stressors due to inadequate resources (eg, physical, psychological, cognitive, or behavioral) (Carpenito, 1997b).

• Related Factors

Family member(s): significant health challenge; chronically unexpressed feelings of guilt, anxiety, hostility, despair; inappropriate coping mechanisms; highly ambivalent relationships; arbitrary handling of resistance to treatment by caregivers; *Caregiver Role Strain.*

• Defining Characteristics

— *SUBJECTIVE DATA* (reported) —

Distorted perception by significant others of client's health problem.

— *OBJECTIVE DATA* (observed) —

Neglectful care, prolonged over concern about family member(s) with health challenge, rejection, abandonment, adherence to usual routine without regard for needs of family member(s), assuming symptoms of client, neglect of self or other family members, decisions detrimental to economic or social well-being, agitation, aggression, dependence or helplessness of significant others.

• Compare With

Caregiver Role Strain; Family Coping: Compromised, Ineffective; Family Processes, Altered; Parental Role Conflict; Parenting, Altered.

Family Coping: Potential for Growth

The state in which family member(s) exhibits desire and readiness for enhanced growth related to ability to manage family member's health care challenges.

• Related Factors

Family experiencing significant health challenge to one or more of its members, another family member ready for self-actualization.

• Defining Characteristics

— *SUBJECTIVE DATA* (reported) —

Growing impact of crisis on personal values, priorities, goals, or relationships; interest in making contact with others in similar situation.

— *OBJECTIVE DATA* (observed) —

Movement toward health-promoting and enriching lifestyle, auditing and negotiating of treatment programs, choice of experiences that optimize wellness.

• Compare With

Therapeutic Regimen.

Individual, Effective Management of; Family Process, Altered: Alcoholism

The state in which the psychosocial, spiritual, and physiologic functions of the family unit are chronically disorganized, leading to conflict, denial of problems, resistance to change, ineffective problem solving, and a series of self-perpetuating crises.

• Related Factors

Abuse of alcohol, family history of alcoholism, resistance to treatment, inadequate coping skills, genetic predisposition, addictive personality, lack of problem-solving skills, biochemical influences.

• Defining Characteristics

— *SUBJECTIVE DATA* (reported) —

Decreased self-esteem, worthlessness, anger/suppressed rage, frustration, powerlessness, anxiety/tension/distress, insecurity, repressed emotions, responsibility for alcoholic's behavior, lingering resentment, shame/embarrassment, guilt, hurt, unhappiness, emotional isolation/loneliness, vulnerability, mistrust, hopelessness, rejection.

— *OBJECTIVE DATA* (observed) —

Expression of anger inappropriately, difficulty with intimate relationships, loss of control of drinking, impaired communication, ineffective problem-solving skills, enabling to maintain drinking, inability to meet emotional needs of its members, manipulation, dependency, criticizing, blaming, alcohol abuse, broken promises, rationalization/denial of problems, refusal to get help/inability to accept and receive help appropriately, blaming, inadequate understanding or knowledge of alcoholism.

• Compare With

Family Coping: Compromised, Ineffective; Family Coping: Disabling, Ineffective; Family Processes, Altered; Coping, Ineffective Individual.

Family Processes, Altered

The state in which a family that normally functions effectively experiences dysfunction.

• Related Factors

Situation transition or crisis, developmental transition or crisis.

• Defining Characteristics

— *SUBJECTIVE DATA* (reported) —

Family unable to express or accept wide range of feelings, unable to express or accept feelings of members.

— *OBJECTIVE DATA* (observed) —

Family members: unable to meet physical, emotional, or spiritual needs; unable to relate to each other for mutual growth and maturation; unable to change or deal with traumatic experience constructively; unable to accept help; uninvolved in community activities; rigidity in functions and roles; absence of respect for individuality and autonomy of each other; failure to accomplish current or past developmental tasks; failure to send and receive clear messages; unhealthy decision-making processes; poor communication of family rules, rituals, symbols; perpetuation of family myths; inappropriate level and direction of energy; parents don't demonstrate respect for each other's views on child-rearing practices.

• Compare With

Family Coping: Compromised, Ineffective; Parental Role Conflict; Parenting, Altered.

Fatigue

An overwhelming, sustained sense of exhaustion and decreased capacity for physical and mental work.

• Related Factors (Etiology)

Decreased or increased metabolic energy production, overwhelming psychological or emotional demands, increased energy requirements to perform activities of daily living, excessive social or role demands, states of discomfort, altered body chemistry (eg, medications, drug withdrawal, chemotherapy), anemia.

• Defining Characteristics

— *SUBJECTIVE DATA* (reported) —

Unremitting and overwhelming lack of energy; inability to maintain usual routines, need for additional energy to accomplish routine tasks; impaired ability to concentrate; decreased libido; disinterest in surroundings or introspection.

— *OBJECTIVE DATA* (observed) —

Emotionally labile or irritable, decreased performance, lethargy or listlessness, increase in physical complaints, accident-prone.

• Compare With

Activity Intolerance; Sleep Pattern Disturbance; Self-Care Deficit.

Fear

The state in which a person experiences a feeling of dread and is able to identify its source(s).

• Related Factors

Actual or perceived threat of pain, disability, disease, physical or psychological discomfort or harm, inability to control situations or cope effectively, loss (of objects, significant others, capabilities, role function, or independence); *Knowledge Deficit.*

• Defining Characteristics

— *SUBJECTIVE DATA* (reported) —

Apprehension, terror, or panic in response to an identifiable source; insomnia; dry mouth; appetite loss.

— *OBJECTIVE DATA* (observed) —

Aggression; irritability; vigilance; increased blood pressure, pulse, and respirations; increased perspiration, pallor, muscle tension; diarrhea, urinary frequency.

• Compare With

Anxiety.

Fluid Volume Deficit

The state in which a person experiences vascular, extracellular, or intracellular dehydration.

• Related Factors

Loss of body fluids (eg, vomiting, diarrhea, GI suction, wound drainage, diaphoresis), decreased fluid intake (eg, nausea, depression, fatigue, lack of access to fluids), fluid shifts (eg, burns, ascites, effusions), fever.

• Defining Characteristics

— *SUBJECTIVE DATA* (reported) —

Dry mouth, thirst, weakness.

— *OBJECTIVE DATA* (observed) —

Weight loss, dry skin and mucous membranes, decreased skin turgor, oliguria, concentrated urine, postural hypotension, weak or rapid pulse, output greater than intake, changes in serum sodium, hemoconcentration.

• Clinical Alert

Report onset of confusion, hypotension, or arrhythmias (may indicate electrolyte imbalance or hypovolemia, which require immediate physician-prescribed interventions).

• Compare With

Fluid Volume Deficit, Risk for.

Fluid Volume Deficit, Risk for

The state in which a person is at risk of experiencing vascular, interstitial, or intracellular dehydration.

• Risk Factors

See related factors for *Fluid Volume Deficit.*

Fluid Volume Excess

The state in which a person experiences increased fluid retention and edema.

• Related Factors

Organ or system disease or immaturity, excess fluid intake, excess sodium intake, decreased plasma protein, side effects of medications, pregnancy.

• Defining Characteristics

— *SUBJECTIVE DATA* (reported) —

Anxiety, shortness of breath, orthopnea, ankle swelling, weight gain.

— *OBJECTIVE DATA* (observed) —

Restlessness; edema; taut, shiny skin; effusion; anasarca; weight gain; intake greater than output; S_3 heart sound; pulmonary congestion on chest x-ray; rales (crackles); change in respiratory pattern; change in mental status; decreased hemoglobin and hematocrit; blood pressure changes; central venous pressure changes; pulmonary artery pressure changes; jugular vein distention; positive hepatojugular reflex; oliguria; specific gravity changes; azotemia; altered electrolytes.

Gas Exchange, Impaired

The state in which a person experiences a decreased passage of oxygen and/or carbon dioxide between the alveoli of the lungs and the vascular system.

• Related Factors

Ventilation or perfusion imbalance, respiratory impairment, acute respiratory failure, altitude sickness, anemia, carbon monoxide poisoning, smoke inhalation.

• Defining Characteristics

— *SUBJECTIVE DATA* (reported) —

Dyspnea, apprehension.

— *OBJECTIVE DATA* (observed) —

Confusion, somnolence, restlessness, irritability, tachypnea, hypercapnia, hypoxemia, rapid heart rate, abnormal arterial blood gasses.

• Clinical Alert

Identifying and treating *Risk for Ineffective Airway Clearance* or *Ineffective Breathing Pattern* is essential to preventing *Impaired Gas Exchange*.

• Compare With

Activity Intolerance; Airway Clearance, Ineffective; Breathing Pattern, Ineffective.

Grieving*

The state in which a person or group experiences a normal pattern of extreme feelings of loss and sadness in response to an actual or perceived loss (of an object, relationship, loved one, pet, capability, body part, body function, or job status).

• Related Factors

Actual or perceived loss.

• Defining Characteristics

— *SUBJECTIVE DATA* (reported) —

During the first year after a loss: sadness in response to loss; guilt; unresolved issues; anger; mood swings; difficulty expressing loss; inability to stop crying, concentrate, make decisions, or participate in meaningful activities or relationships.

— *OBJECTIVE DATA* (observed) —

During the first year after a loss: idealization of lost object or person; changes in eating habits, activity level, libido, sleep or dream patterns; reliving of past experiences; interference with life functions; regression; labile affect; decreased ability to concentrate or pursue tasks.

*Not on the list as of 1997; added by author.

• Compare With

Coping, Ineffective Individual; Grieving, Anticipatory; Grieving, Dysfunctional; Spiritual Distress.

Grieving, Anticipatory

The state in which a person or family experiences feelings of anxiety, fear, or sadness in response to a possible loss (of object, relationship, loved one, pet, capability, body part, body function, or job status).

• Related Factors

Anticipated loss.

• Defining Characteristics

— *SUBJECTIVE DATA* (reported) —

Distress at potential loss, guilt, anger, sorrow; denial of potential loss.

— *OBJECTIVE DATA* (observed) —

Change in eating habits, sleep patterns, activity level, libido, communication patterns.

• Compare With

Grieving; Grieving, Dysfunctional; Spiritual Distress.

Grieving, Dysfunctional

The state in which a person or group experiences prolonged and exaggerated feelings of loss and sadness in response to an actual or perceived loss (of an object, loved one, pet, capability, relationship, or body part).

• Related Factors

Actual or perceived loss.

• Defining Characteristics

— *SUBJECTIVE DATA* (reported) —

More than a year after a loss: inability to participate in meaningful activities or relationships because of symptoms associated with sadness over loss (see defining characteristics of *Grieving*).

— *OBJECTIVE DATA* (observed) —

More than a year after a loss: inability to participate in meaningful activities or relationships because of symptoms associated with sadness over loss (see defining characteristics of *Grieving*).

• Compare With

Coping, Ineffective Individual; Grieving; Grieving, Anticipatory; Spiritual Distress.

Growth and Development, Altered

The state in which a child's growth or development is below the norm for his or her age group.

• Related Factors

Inadequate caregiving (eg, indifference, neglect, abuse, inconsistent responsiveness, multiple caregivers), separation from significant others, environmental and stimulation deficiencies, physical illness or disability, prescribed dependence.

• Defining Characteristics

— *OBJECTIVE DATA* (observed) —

Delay or difficulty in performing skills (motor, social, or expressive) typical of age group; altered physical growth; inability to perform self-care or self-control activities appropriate for age; regression in previously acquired skills; flat affect, listlessness, decreased responses.

Health Maintenance, Altered

The state in which a person (or group) experiences or is at risk of experiencing a disruption in health because of an unhealthy lifestyle. (Carpenito, 1997a)

• Related Factors

Decreased communication skills (written, verbal, nonverbal), inability to make valid judgments, perceptual or cognitive impairment (complete or partial lack of gross or fine motor skills), developmental delay, inadequate coping skills, lack of resources, unavailable or inadequate support system, poor health habits.

• Defining Characteristics

— *SUBJECTIVE DATA* (reported) —

Interest in improving health behaviors.

— *OBJECTIVE DATA* (observed) —

Lack of knowledge regarding basic health practices, lack of adaptive behaviors to internal or external environmental changes, inability to take responsibility for meeting basic health practices in any or all functional patterns, failure to seek basic health information.

• Compare With

Coping, Ineffective Individual; Knowledge Deficit; Management of Therapeutic Regimen, Ineffective Individual.

Health-Seeking Behaviors (Specify)

A state in which a person in stable health is actively seeking ways to change health habits or the environment to move toward a higher level of health.

• Related Factors

Ability to meet basic health needs, achievement of age-appropriate illness prevention measures, good or excellent health, desire to enhance current health status or practices.

• Defining Characteristics

— *SUBJECTIVE DATA* (reported) —

Desire to seek higher level of wellness or increase control of health practices, concern about the effect of current environmental conditions on health status.

— *OBJECTIVE DATA* (observed) —

Unfamiliarity with wellness community resources, behaviors not consistent with health promotion.

Home Maintenance Management, Impaired

The state in which a person or family is unable to maintain a safe, growth-promoting environment independently.

• Related Factors

Individual or family member disease or injury; insufficient organization or planning; insufficient finances; unfamiliarity with available resources; impaired cognitive or emotional functioning; lack of knowledge, role models, or support systems; young children in home.

• Defining Characteristics

— *SUBJECTIVE DATA* (reported) —

Difficulty in maintaining home in a comfortable fashion, seeking of assistance with home maintenance, outstanding debts or financial crises, history of accidents.

— *OBJECTIVE DATA* (observed) —

Disorderly surroundings; unwashed or unavailable cooking equipment, clothes, or linen; accumulated dirt, food wastes, or unhygienic wastes; offensive odors; inappropriate household temperature; overtaxed family members (eg, exhausted, anxious); lack of necessary equipment or aids; presence of vermin or rodents; repeated hygienic disorders, infestations, or infections; hazards in the home.

• Compare With

Injury, Risk for.

Hopelessness

A state in which a person sees limited or no alternatives or acceptable choices and is unable to mobilize energy on his or her own behalf.

• Related Factors

Prolonged activity restriction creating isolation, failing or deteriorating physiologic condition, long-term stress, abandonment, lost belief in transcendent values or God.

• Defining Characteristics

— *SUBJECTIVE DATA* (reported) —

Inability to make choices, solve problems, or perform activity; apathy; indifference; decreased appetite.

— *OBJECTIVE DATA* (observed) —

Passive anger, flat affect, sighing, decreased response to stimuli, decreased verbalization, turning away from speaker, closing eyes or shrugging in response to speaker, decreased or increased sleep, lack of initiative, lack of involvement in care or passively allowing care.

• Compare With

Powerlessness; Spiritual Distress.

Hyperthermia

A state in which body temperature is elevated above normal range.

• Related Factors

Heat exposure, vigorous activity, medications or anesthesia, inappropriate clothing, increased metabolic rate, illness or trauma, dehydration, decreased ability to perspire.

• Defining Characteristics

— *OBJECTIVE DATA* (observed) —

Increased body temperature above normal range, flushed or warm skin, increased respiratory rate, tachycardia, malaise, irritability, seizures or convulsions.

• Clinical Alert

Immediately report temperature elevations associated with a shaking chill, hypotension, or confusion, which may indicate onset of septic shock. Also report frequent unexplained elevations, sustained elevations, or elevations accompanied by symptoms of infection.

• Compare With

Body Temperature, Risk for Altered; Thermoregulation, Ineffective.

Hypothermia

The state in which a person's body temperature is reduced below 95°F.

• Related Factors

Exposure to cold, inadequate clothing, evaporation of moisture from skin, illness or trauma, damage to hypothalamus, inability or decreased ability to shiver, medications causing vasodilation, alcohol consumption, malnutrition, decreased metabolic rate, inactivity, aging, neonatal period, prematurity.

• Defining Characteristics

— *SUBJECTIVE DATA* (reported) —

Sensation of feeling cold.

— *OBJECTIVE DATA* (observed) —

Body temperature below normal range, shivering, cool skin, pallor, confusion, slow capillary refill, tachycardia, cyanotic nail beds, hypertension, piloerection.

• Compare With

Body Temperature, Risk for Altered; Thermoregulation, Ineffective.

Infant Behavior, Disorganized

The state in which an infant experiences an alteration in integration and modulation of the physiologic and behavioral systems of functioning (ie, autonomic, motor, state, organizational, self-regulatory and attentional-interactional systems).

• Related Factors

Pain, oral/motor problems, feeding intolerance, environmental overstimulation, lack of containment/boundaries, prematurity, invasive/painful procedures.

• Defining Characteristics

— *OBJECTIVE DATA* (observed) —

Change from baseline physiologic measures, tremors, startles, twitches, hyperextension of arms and legs, diffuse/unclear sleep, deficient self-regulatory behaviors, deficient response to visual/auditory stimuli, yawning, apnea.

Infant Behavior, Disorganized, Risk for

The state in which an infant is at risk for alteration in integration and modulation of the physiologic and behavioral systems of functioning (ie, autonomic, motor, state, organizational, self-regulatory, and attentional-interactional systems).

• Risk Factors

See related factors for *Infant Behavior, Disorganized.*

Infant Behavior, Organized, Potential for Enhanced

A state in which the pattern of modulation of the physiologic and behavioral systems of functioning of an infant (ie, autonomic, motor, state, organizational, self-regulatory, and attentional-interactional systems) is satisfactory but can be improved, resulting in higher levels of integration in response to environmental stimuli.

• Related Factors

Prematurity, Pain.

• Defining Characteristics

— *OBJECTIVE DATA* (observed) —

Stable physiologic measures, definite sleep–wake states, use of some self-regulatory behaviors, response to visual/auditory stimuli.

Infant Feeding Pattern, Ineffective

A state in which an infant demonstrates an impaired ability to suck or to coordinate the suck–swallow response.

• Related Factors

Prematurity, neurologic impairment or delay, oral hypersensitivity, prolonged NPO, anatomic abnormality.

• Defining Characteristics

— *OBJECTIVE DATA* (observed) —

Inability to initiate or sustain an effective suck; inability to coordinate sucking, swallowing, and breathing; coughing or choking with feeding.

• Compare With

Aspiration, Risk for; Breastfeeding, Ineffective.

Infection, Risk for

The state in which a person is at increased risk for being invaded by pathogenic organisms.

• Risk Factors

Inadequate primary defenses (broken skin, traumatized tissue, decreased ciliary action, stasis of body fluids, change in pH of secretions, altered peristalsis); inadequate secondary defenses (decreased hemoglobin, leukopenia, suppressed inflammatory response); immunosuppression; inadequate acquired immunity; chronic disease; malnutrition; environmental hazards (work, travel); treatment-related hazards (invasive lines or procedures, surgery, medications); extremes of age; *Knowledge Deficit (self-protection);* high-risk behaviors (eg, unsafe sex, drug abuse).

• Compare With

Protection, Altered.

Injury, Risk for

The state in which a person is at risk for injury as a result of individual risk factors or environmental hazards.

• Risk Factors

Individual: extremes of age, deconditioned state, difficulty ambulating, lack of knowledge of hazards, altered mental status, history of frequent falls, *Sensory-Perceptual Alterations.*
Environmental: workplace hazards without adequate safety precautions (eg, hard-hats, protective goggles); steps in poor repair, poor lighting, lack of handrails or side rails; *Impaired Home Maintenance Management.*

• Compare With

Aspiration, Risk for; Poisoning, Risk for; Suffocation, Risk for; Trauma, Risk for; Home Maintenance Management, Impaired.

Knowledge Deficit (Specify)

The state in which a person lacks the skills or information to successfully manage his or her own health care.

• Related Factors

Cognitive limitation, lack of recall, lack of previous opportunity to learn, misinterpretation of information, lack of interest or motivation, unfamiliarity with information sources, inability to read or lack of access to written information, *Fear, Ineffective Denial.*

• Defining Characteristics

— *SUBJECTIVE DATA* (reported) —

Information seeking, dissatisfaction with ability to manage health care, incomplete or inaccurate information related to health care needs, difficulty performing skills.

— *OBJECTIVE DATA* (observed) —

Inaccurate demonstration of skill, behavior inconsistent with instruction, inappropriate or exaggerated behaviors (eg, hysteria, hostility, agitation, apathy).

Loneliness, Risk for

A subjective state in which an individual is at risk for experiencing vague dysphoria.

• Risk Factors

Affectional deprivation, physical isolation, emotional/attentional deprivation, social isolation.

• Compare With

Relocation Stress Syndrome; Social Isolation.

Mobility, Impaired Physical

A state in which a person experiences a limitation of ability for independent movement.

• Related Factors

Intolerance to activity or decreased strength and endurance; pain or discomfort; neuromuscular or musculoskeletal impairment; imposed restrictions of movement, medical protocol.

• Defining Characteristics

— *SUBJECTIVE DATA* (reported) —

Reluctance to attempt movement, pain with movement.

— *OBJECTIVE DATA* (observed) —

Inability to move purposefully (confinement to bed; problems with transfer, ambulation, limited range of motion; decreased muscle strength, control, or mass).

• Author's Note

This diagnosis is appropriate when interventions are aimed at increasing strength and endurance, restoring function, or preventing deterioration.

• Compare With

Activity Intolerance; Disuse Syndrome, Risk for; Self-Care Deficit.

Noncompliance (Specify)

The state in which a person expresses an informed decision not to adhere to a therapeutic recommendation, which may significantly compromise health status (see author's note below).

• Related Factors

Undesirable treatment side effects; previous unsuccessful experience with health regimens, lack of motivation and trust, spiritual/cultural values.

• Defining Characteristics

— *SUBJECTIVE DATA* (reported) —

Decision not to adhere to therapeutic recommendation in spite of knowledge of possible consequences.

— *OBJECTIVE DATA* (observed) —

Behavior inconsistent with therapeutic recommendation, development of complications, exacerbation of symptoms, failure to make progress toward recovery, failure to keep or make appointments.

• Author's Note

This diagnosis is poorly developed. The right of an informed, responsible adult to choose not to comply with a therapeutic recommendation must be respected. More appropriate diagnoses to consider are listed below.

• Compare With

Coping, Ineffective Individual; Denial, Ineffective; Family Coping: Disabling, Ineffective; Knowledge Deficit; Therapeutic Regimen: Individual, Ineffective Management of; Spiritual Distress.

Memory, Impaired

The state in which an individual experiences the inability to remember or recall bits of information or behavioral skills. Impaired memory may be attributed to pathophysiologic or situational causes that are either temporary or permanent.

• Related Factors

Acute or chronic hypoxia, anemia, decreased cardiac output, fluid and electrolyte imbalance, neurologic disturbances, excessive environmental disturbances.

• Defining Characteristics

— *SUBJECTIVE DATA* (reported) —

Reported experiences of forgetting, inability to recall recent or past events.

— *OBJECTIVE DATA* (observed) —

Observed experiences of forgetting, inability to determine if a behavior was performed, inability to learn or retain new skills or information, inability to perform a previously learned skill, inability to recall factual information.

• Compare With

Confusion, Chronic; Thought Processes, Altered.

Nutrition, Altered: Less than Body Requirements

The state in which a person experiences an inability to ingest, digest, or absorb sufficient nutrients to meet metabolic needs.

• Related Factors

Poor appetite, stomatitis, dysphagia, poorly fitting dentures, fad dieting, poor food choices, inability to obtain or prepare food (eg, physical or financial limitations), eating disorders (eg, anorexia nervosa, bulimia), increased metabolic requirements (eg, burns, infection, cancer), absorption disorders (eg, Crohn's disease, cystic fibrosis), medication side effects.

• Defining Characteristics

— *SUBJECTIVE DATA* (reported) —

Poor appetite; aversion to eating; lack of interest in food; altered taste sensation; satiety immediately after ingesting small amount of food; abdominal pain with or without pathology; abdominal cramping; frequent purging; perceived inability to ingest food; lack of information, misinformation; misconceptions regarding nutritional requirements.

— *OBJECTIVE DATA* (observed) —

Food intake calculated to be less than metabolic requirements; body weight 20% below ideal; decreased serum albumin, muscle mass or tone, subcutaneous fat; pale conjunctival and mucous membranes; excessive hair loss; weight inconsistent with perception of being fat.

• Compare With

Oral Mucous Membrane, Altered; Self-Care Deficit, Feeding; Home Maintenance Management, Impaired; Swallowing, Impaired; Infant Feeding Pattern, Ineffective.

Nutrition, Altered: More than Body Requirements

The state in which a person is experiencing an intake of nutrients in excess of metabolic needs.

• Related Factors

Obesity in one or both parents; rapid transition across growth percentiles during infancy and childhood; use of solid food as major food source before 5 months of age; use of food as reward or comfort measure; frequent, closely spaced pregnancies; higher baseline weight at beginning of each pregnancy; inadequate exercise or activity patterns; poor dietary habits (eg, snacking; unbalanced meals; high fat content foods); lack of knowledge of nutritional value of food; dysfunctional eating patterns; disease (thyroid problems, diabetes); medication side effects (eg, steroids, birth control pills).

• Defining Characteristics

— *SUBJECTIVE DATA* (reported) —

Eating in response to external cues such as time of day, social situation; eating in response to internal cues other than hunger (eg, *Anxiety*).

— *OBJECTIVE DATA* (observed) —

Excessive intake in relation to metabolic need; weight 20% over ideal for height and frame; triceps skin fold greater than 15 mm in men, 25 mm in women; percentage of body fat greater than that recommended based on age and sex; pairing food with other activities; concentrating food intake at end of day.

• Compare With

Altered Nutrition: Risk for More than Body Requirements; Coping, Ineffective Individual.

Nutrition, Altered: Risk for More than Body Requirements

The state in which a person is at risk of experiencing an intake of nutrients in excess of metabolic needs.

• Risk Factors

See related factors for *Nutrition, Altered: More than Body Requirements.*

Oral Mucous Membrane, Altered

The state in which a person experiences disruptions in the tissue layers of the oral cavity.

• Related Factors

Radiation to head or neck, oral surgery, periodontal disease, chemical irritants (eg, alcohol, tobacco, drugs), dehydration, ill-fitting dentures or braces, carious teeth, presence of endotracheal or nasogastric tube, NPO for more than 24 hours, ineffective oral hygiene, mouth breathing, malnutrition, infection, absent or decreased salivation, medication side effects (chemotherapy, immunosuppressants).

• Defining Characteristics

— *SUBJECTIVE DATA* (reported) —

Oral pain or discomfort.

— *OBJECTIVE DATA* (observed) —

Coated tongue, stomatitis, lesions or ulcers, leukoplakia, edema, hyperemia, plaque, vesicles, hemorrhagic gingivitis, halitosis.

• Compare With

Tissue Integrity, Impaired.

Pain

A state in which a person experiences and reports the presence of severe discomfort or an uncomfortable sensation.

• Related Factors

Injuring agents (biologic, chemical, physical, psychological), problems with structure or function of organ or systems, drug tolerance.

• Defining Characteristics

— *SUBJECTIVE DATA* (reported) —

Description of pain or discomfort.

— *OBJECTIVE DATA* (observed) —

Guarding or protective behavior; self-focusing; narrowed focus (altered time perception, withdrawal from social contact, impaired thought process); distraction behavior (moaning, crying, pacing, seeking out other people or activities, restlessness); facial mask of pain (eyes lack luster, beaten look, fixed or scattered movement, grimace); altered muscle tone, autonomic responses (diaphoresis, blood pressure and pulse changes, pupillary dilation, changes in respiratory rate).

• Clinical Alert

Report new onset of pain or unrelieved pain. Recognize that there are national guidelines for pain management available from the Department of Human Services.

• Compare With

Pain, Chronic.

Pain, Chronic

A state in which a person experiences pain that continues for more than 6 months in duration.

• Related Factors

Chronic physical or psychosocial disability, depression, problems with organ or system structure or function, drug tolerance.

• Defining Characteristics

— *SUBJECTIVE DATA* (reported) —

Pain for more than 6 months; fear of reinjury; altered ability to continue previous activities; poor appetite; changes in weight, behavior, or sleep patterns; depression, frustration, anger; *Hopelessness*.

— *OBJECTIVE DATA* (observed) —

Behavior changes, facial mask, guarded movement.

• Clinical Alert

People with *Chronic Pain* may not demonstrate usual autonomic response associated with pain (increased pulse and blood pressure). They may also appear to be pain-free (eg, smiling, laughing), however, this is usually a result of efforts to overcome pain through distraction, and should not be considered a sign that the person really isn't in pain.

• Compare With

Pain.

Parental Role Conflict

The state in which a parent experiences role confusion and conflict in response to crisis.

• Related Factors

Separation from child, invasive or restrictive modalities (eg, isolation, intubation), specialized care center policies, home care of a child with special needs (eg, apnea monitoring, postural drainage, hyperalimentation), change in marital status, interruptions of family life due to home-care regimen, *Caregiver Role Strain*.

• Defining Characteristics

— *SUBJECTIVE DATA* (reported) —

Concern or feeling of inadequacy or reluctance to provide for child's physical and emotional needs; concerns about changes in parental role or family functioning, communication, or health; actual or perceived loss of control over decisions related to child (or children).

— *OBJECTIVE DATA* (observed) —

Disruption in care routines; reluctance to participate in usual care activities, even with encouragement and support.

• Compare With

Caregiver Role Strain; Family Coping: Disabling, Ineffective; Family Processes, Altered; Parenting, Altered.

Parent/Infant/Child Attachment, Risk for Altered

A state in which there is a risk for disruption of the interactive process between parent/significant other and infant that fosters the development of a protective and nurturing reciprocal relationship.

• Risk Factors

Inability of parents to meet the personal needs anxiety associated with the parent role, substance abuse, premature infant, ill infant/child who is unable to effectively initiate parental contact due to altered behavioral organization, separation, physical barriers, lack of privacy.

• Compare With

Infant Behavior, Disorganized; Parental Role Conflict.

Parenting, Altered

The state in which parent figure(s) experiences inability to create an environment that promotes the optimum growth and development of a child or children.

• Related Factors

Parent figure(s): lack of (or ineffective) role model, physical and psychosocial abuse, lack of support from significant other, unmet social or emotional needs, multiple pregnancies, lack of knowledge, *Caregiver Role Strain.*
Parent figure(s) or child(ren): actual or perceived threat to physical or emotional survival, unrealistic expectations, introduction of new family member(s) (eg, birth, adoption), mental or physical illness, stress.
Child(ren): absent or inappropriate response.

• Defining Characteristics

— *SUBJECTIVE DATA* (reported) —

Inability to control child, disappointment in gender or physical characteristics of child, resentment toward child, disgust at body functions of child, feeling of inadequacy.

— *OBJECTIVE DATA* (observed) —

Parental abandonment, child abuse or neglect, runaway child, absence of parental attachment, failure to make or keep appointments with health care providers, inattention to needs of child, inappropriate caregiving behaviors, inappropriate or inconsistent disciplinary measures, frequent accidents or illnesses, delay in growth and development of child (children).

• Compare With

Caregiver Role Strain; Family Coping: Disabling, Ineffective; Family Processes, Altered; Growth and Development, Altered; Infant Behavior, Disorganized; Parental Role Conflict.

Parenting, Risk for Altered

The state in which parent figure(s) is at risk for experiencing inability to create an environment that promotes optimum growth and development of a child or children.

• Risk Factors

See related factors of *Altered Parenting.*

• Compare With

Caregiver Role Strain; Family Coping: Disabling, Ineffective; Family Processes, Altered; Growth and Development, Altered; Infant Behavior, Disorganized; Parental Role Conflict.

Perioperative Positioning Injury, Risk for

A state in which the client is at risk for injury as a result of the environmental conditions found in the perioperative setting.

• Risk Factors

Disorientation, immobilization, muscle weakness, sensory/perceptual disturbances due to anesthesia, obesity, emaciation, edema.

Peripheral Neurovascular Dysfunction, Risk for

A state in which a person is at risk of experiencing a disruption in circulation, sensation, or motion of an extremity.

• Risk Factors

Fractures, trauma, burns, vascular obstruction, immobilization, orthopedic surgery, mechanical compression (eg, tourniquet, cast, brace, dressing, or restraint).

• Clinical Alert

Report deviations from baseline neurovascular assessment findings that don't respond to nurse-prescribed interventions immediately so that measures can be taken to prevent irreversible neuromuscular damage.

• Compare With

Tissue Perfusion, Altered (peripheral).

Personal Identity Disturbance

The state in which a person experiences an inability to distinguish between self and nonself.

• Author's Note

No defining characteristics or related factors listed by NANDA. This diagnosis was accepted for study in 1978, but hasn't been developed sufficiently to be clinically useful.

Poisoning, Risk for

The state in which a person is at risk of accidental exposure to (or ingestion of) drugs or dangerous substances in doses sufficient to cause toxicity.

• Risk Factors

Individual: reduced vision, occupational setting without adequate safeguards, lack of safety or drug education or precautions, cognitive or emotional difficulties, insufficient finances.
Environmental: large supplies of drugs in house; medicines or potential poisons (cleansers and so forth) stored in unlocked cabinets accessible to children or confused persons; availability of illicit drugs; flaking, peeling paint or plaster in presence of young children; chemical contamination of food and water; unprotected contact with heavy metals or chemicals; paint, lacquer, and other materials with volatile solvents in poorly ventilated areas or without effective protection; poisonous vegetation; atmospheric pollutants.

• Compare With

Home Maintenance Management, Impaired.

Post-Trauma Response

The state in which a person experiences a sustained, painful response to unexpected, extraordinary life event(s).

• Related Factors

Disasters, wars, epidemics, rape, assault, torture, catastrophic illness or accident.

• Defining Characteristics

— *SUBJECTIVE DATA* (reported) —

Reexperience of the traumatic event that may be identified in cognitive, affective, or sensory motor activities (eg, flashbacks, intrusive thoughts, repetitive dreams or nightmares, excessive verbalization of the traumatic event, survival guilt or guilt about behavior required for survival). Psychic or emotional numbness (impaired interpretation of reality, confusion, dissociation, amnesia, vagueness about traumatic event).

— *OBJECTIVE DATA* (observed) —

Altered lifestyle: self-destructiveness, such as substance abuse, suicide attempt, or other acting-out behavior, difficulty with interpersonal relationships, phobia regarding trauma, poor impulse control, irritability and explosiveness; constricted affect.

• Compare With

Rape Trauma Syndrome.

Powerlessness

The state in which a person perceives a personal lack of control over certain events or situations that impact on outlook, goals, and lifestyle (Carpenito, 1997a).

• Related Factors

Illness-related regimen, inability to perform self-care; health care environment or routines, interpersonal interactions, previous lifestyle of maintaining or enjoying control.

• Defining Characteristics

— *SUBJECTIVE DATA* (reported) —

Lack of control or influence over a situation or outcome, continued illness or deterioration despite compliance with prescribed regimen, anger.

— *OBJECTIVE DATA* (observed) —

Irritability, aggression, violent behavior, lack of cooperation with planned care, unwillingness to seek information regarding health status.

• Compare With

Hopelessness.

Protection, Altered

The state in which a person experiences a decrease in the ability to guard the self from internal or external threats such as illness or injury.

• Related Factors

Extremes of age; inadequate nutrition; alcohol abuse; abnormal blood profiles (leukopenia, thrombocytopenia, anemia, coagulation); drug therapies (antineoplastics, corticosteroids, immunosuppressants, anticoagulants, thrombolytics); treatments (surgery, radiation); diseases such as cancer, diabetes, and immune disorders.

• Defining Characteristics

— *SUBJECTIVE DATA* (reported) —

Dyspnea, itching, fatigue, anorexia, frequent illnesses, insomnia, *Activity Intolerance.*

— *OBJECTIVE DATA* (observed) —

Deficient immunity, impaired healing, altered clotting, maladaptive stress response, neurosensory alteration, chilling, perspiring, cough, restlessness, weakness, immobility, disorientation, pressure sores.

• Compare With

Infection, Risk for; Injury, Risk for.

Rape Trauma Syndrome*

The state in which a person experiences actual or attempted sexual penetration (vaginal, anal, oral) against his or her will or consent, resulting in an acute phase of disorganization of lifestyle and a long-term process of reorganization.

• Related Factors

Attempted or actual sexual assault.

• Defining Characteristics

— *SUBJECTIVE DATA* (reported) —

Emotional reactions (anger, fear, embarrassment, humiliation, self-blame, desire for revenge); GI symptoms (nausea, vomiting, anorexia); genitourinary discomfort (pain, tenderness); muscle tension; insomnia; nightmares; changes in sexual behavior, relationship with opposite sex, or lifestyle; *Anxiety; Fear.*

— *OBJECTIVE DATA* (observed) —

Changes in behavior, communication patterns, appearance, or lifestyle; reactivation of previous conditions (physical illness, psychiatric illness, alcohol or drug abuse). *Additional data for Silent Reaction:* lack of verbalization of the occurrence of rape.

• Clinical Alert

Referral of this diagnosis to a professional qualified in rape counseling is likely to result in improved outcomes.

*NANDA has this listed as three different diagnoses (*Rape Trauma Syndrome, Rape Trauma Syndrome: Silent Reaction, Rape Trauma Syndrome: Compound Reaction*), all with the same definition.

Relocation Stress Syndrome

The state in which a person experiences physiologic or psychosocial disturbances as a result of transfer from one environment to another.

• Related Factors

Past, concurrent, or recent losses; losses involved with decision to move; little or no preparation for the move; moderate to high degree of environmental change; history and types of previous transfers; feeling of powerlessness; lack of adequate support system; impaired psychosocial or physical health status; advanced age.

• Defining Characteristics

— *SUBJECTIVE DATA* (reported) —

Apprehension, increased confusion (elderly population), depression, loneliness, concern about or unwillingness to transfer, increased verbalization of needs, insecurity, lack of trust, unfavorable comparison of post- to pre-transfer staff, anger, *Anxiety.*

— *OBJECTIVE DATA* (observed) —

Change in eating habits or weight, sleep disturbances, GI disturbances, dependency, restlessness, sad affect, vigilance, withdrawal.

• Compare With

Loneliness; Powerlessness; Social Isolation.

Role Performance, Altered

The state in which a person perceives a disruption in ability to perform usual roles.

• Related Factors

Change in capacity to resume role, lack of knowledge of role, change in usual patterns of responsibility.

• Defining Characteristics

— *SUBJECTIVE DATA* (reported) —

Change in self-perception of role, role conflict.

— *OBJECTIVE DATA* (observed) —

Change in others' perception of role.

• Compare With

Adjustment, Impaired; Parental Role Conflict; Sexuality Patterns, Altered; Home Maintenance Management, Impaired.

Self-Care Deficit, Bathing/Hygiene*

A state in which a person experiences an impaired ability to perform or complete bathing or hygiene activities for oneself.

• Related Factors

Decreased mobility, strength, or endurance: pain, discomfort; perceptual, cognitive, neuromuscular, or musculoskeletal impairment; depression; *Anxiety* (severe); *Activity Intolerance.*

• Defining Characteristics

— *OBJECTIVE DATA* (observed) —

Inability to: wash body parts, obtain (or get to) water, regulate temperature or flow.

• Compare With

Activity Intolerance; Mobility, Impaired Physical.

Self-Care Deficit, Feeding*

A state in which a person experiences an impaired ability to perform or complete feeding activities for oneself.

• Related Factors

Decreased mobility, strength, or endurance; pain, discomfort; perceptual, cognitive neuromuscular, or musculoskeletal impairment; depression; *Anxiety* (severe); *Activity Intolerance.*

• Defining Characteristics

— *OBJECTIVE DATA*—

Inability to bring food from a receptacle to the mouth.

• Compare With

Mobility, Impaired Physical; Activity Intolerance; Nutrition, Altered: Less than Body Requirements.

Self-Care Deficit, Dressing/Grooming*

A state in which a person experiences an impaired ability to perform or complete dressing and grooming activities for oneself.

• Related Factors

Decreased mobility, strength, or endurance; pain, discomfort; perceptual, cognitive, neuromuscular, or musculoskeletal impairment; depression; *Anxiety* (severe); *Activity Intolerance.*

• Defining Characteristics

— *OBJECTIVE DATA* (observed) —

Impaired ability to: put on or take off necessary items of clothing, obtain or replace articles of clothing, fasten clothing, maintain satisfactory appearance.

• Compare With

Activity Intolerance; Mobility, Impaired Physical.

Self-Care Deficit, Toileting*

A state in which a person experiences an impaired ability to perform or complete toileting activities for oneself.

• Related Factors

Decreased mobility, strength, or endurance; pain, discomfort; perceptual, cognitive, neuromuscular, or musculoskeletal impairment; depression; *Anxiety* (severe); *Activity Intolerance.*

— *OBJECTIVE DATA* (observed) —

Inability to: get to toilet, sit on or rise from toilet; manipulate clothing for toileting, carry out toilet hygiene, flush toilet or empty commode.

• Compare With

Activity Intolerance; Mobility, Impaired Physical.

Self-Esteem Disturbance

The state in which a person experiences negative evaluation or feelings about self or about personal capabilities.

• Related Factors

Relationships characterized by abuse (verbal, sexual, physical), parental neglect, helplessness.

• Defining Characteristics

— *SUBJECTIVE DATA* (reported) —

Shame or guilt; inability to deal with events; rejection of positive feedback or exaggeration of negative feed-

---

*Classsify functional level by using the following code: (0) completely independent; (1) requires use of equipment or device; (2) requires help from another person for assistance, supervision, or teaching; (3) requires help from another person and equipment or device; (4) dependent, doesn't participate in activity.

back; hesitance to try new things or situations; lack of success in relationships, work, or other life events; difficulty making decisions.

— *OBJECTIVE DATA* (observed) —

Dependence on others' opinions; poor eye contact; nonassertive, passive, or indecisive behaviors; excessive seeking of reassurance; overconformance; self-negating verbalization; difficulty making decisions.

• Compare With

Adjustment, Impaired; Coping, Ineffective Individual; Self-Esteem, Situational Low; Self-Esteem, Chronic Low.

Self-Esteem, Chronic Low

The state in which a person experiences long-standing negative evaluation of self or personal capabilities.

• Related Factors

History of ineffective or abusive relationships; unrealistic expectations of child by parent, of parent by child, or of self; inadequate support; rejection or separation; inconsistent punishment; lack of stimulation; restriction of activity; inability to trust significant other.

• Defining Characteristics

— *SUBJECTIVE DATA* (reported) —

Long-standing or chronic symptoms of low self-esteem (see subjective data listed under defining characteristics of *Self-Esteem Disturbance*).

— *OBJECTIVE DATA* (observed) —

Long-standing or chronic signs of low self-esteem (see objective data listed under defining characteristics of *Self-Esteem Disturbance*).

• Compare With

Self-Esteem, Situational Low; Self-Esteem Disturbance.

Self-Esteem, Situational Low

The state in which a person who previously had a positive self-evaluation experiences negative self-evaluation or feelings in response to a loss or change.

• Related Factors

Unemployment, financial problems, divorce, legal difficulties, institutionalization, failure in school or work, hospitalization.

• Defining Characteristics

— *SUBJECTIVE DATA* (reported) —

Episodic occurrence of symptoms of low self-esteem in response to a loss or change (see subjective data listed under defining characteristics of *Self-Esteem Disturbance*).

— *OBJECTIVE DATA* (observed) —

Episodic occurrence of signs of low self-esteem in response to a loss or change (see defining characteristics of *Self-Esteem Disturbance*).

• Compare With

Adjustment, Impaired; Coping, Ineffective Individual; Self-Esteem, Chronic Low; Self-Esteem Disturbance.

Self-Mutilation, Risk for

A state in which a person is at risk of performing an act upon the self to injure, not kill, which produces tissue damage and tension relief.

• Risk Factors

Borderline personality disorder (especially females 16 to 25 years of age); psychotic state (frequently males in young adulthood); emotionally disturbed or battered children; mentally retarded and autistic children; history of self-injury; history of physical, emotional, or sexual abuse; inability to cope with increased psychological or physiologic tension; feelings of depression, rejection, self-hatred, separation anxiety, guilt, and depersonalization; fluctuating emotions; command hallucinations; need for sensory stimuli; parental or emotional deprivation; dysfunctional family.

Sensory–Perceptual Alterations (Specify: visual, auditory, kinesthetic, gustatory, tactile, olfactory)

A state in which a person experiences a change in the amount or pattern of incoming stimuli accompanied by a diminished, exaggerated, distorted, or impaired response to these stimuli.

• Related Factors

Sensory organ deficits; altered sensory reception, transmission, or integration; excessive or insufficient environmental stimuli; sleep deprivation; metabolic alterations (eg, fluid and electrolyte imbalance, acidosis, alkalosis); medication side effects; *Pain;* stress.

• Defining Characteristics

— *SUBJECTIVE DATA* (reported) —

Hallucinations, *Fatigue, Anxiety.*

— *OBJECTIVE DATA* (observed) —

Disorientation to time, place, or person; measurable alteration in sensory acuity; change in behavior or communication pattern; inability to solve problems; inappropriate responses; apathy; restlessness; irritability.

• Compare With

Thought Processes, Altered.

Sexual Dysfunction

The state in which a person experiences a change in sexual function that is viewed as unsatisfying, unrewarding, or inadequate.

• Related Factors

Biopsychosocial alteration of sexuality, ineffectual or absent role models, physical or psychosocial abuse (eg, harmful relationships), vulnerability, values conflict, lack of privacy, lack of significant other, altered body structure or function (eg, pregnancy, recent childbirth, drugs, surgery, anomalies, disease process, trauma, radiation), misinformation or lack of knowledge.

• Defining Characteristics

— *SUBJECTIVE DATA* (reported) —

Problem with sexual function, dissatisfaction with sex role, limitations imposed by disease or therapy, inability to achieve desired sexual satisfaction; seeking of confirmation of desirability, altered relationship with significant other, change of interest in self or others.

— *OBJECTIVE DATA* (observed) —

Frequent sex-related questions.

• Compare With

Sexuality Patterns, Altered.

Sexuality Patterns, Altered

The state in which a person experiences, or is at risk for experiencing, a change in sexual patterns.

• Related Factors

Knowledge or skill deficit about alternative responses to health-related transitions, altered body function or structure, illness or medical treatment; lack of privacy; lack of significant other; ineffective or absent role models; conflicts with sexual orientation or variant preferences; fear of pregnancy or of acquiring or transmitting a sexually transmitted disease; impaired relationship with a significant other.

• Defining Characteristics

— *SUBJECTIVE DATA* (reported) —

Difficulties, limitations, or changes in sexual behaviors or activities.

— *OBJECTIVE DATA* (observed) —

Frequent sex-related questions.

• Compare With

Sexual Dysfunction.

Skin Integrity, Impaired

A state in which a person's skin is altered adversely.

• Related Factors

External factors: extremes of temperature, humidity, chemical substances, secretions or excretions, mechanical factors (shearing forces, pressure, restraints), trauma, radiation, immobilization.
Internal factors: altered nutritional state (obesity, malnutrition), metabolic state, circulation, pigmentation, or skin turgor; impaired sensation; skeletal prominence; developmental factors; immunologic deficits; medication side effects; edema; subcutaneous fat loss; decreased skin turgor.

• Defining Characteristics

— *SUBJECTIVE DATA* (reported) —

Itching, pain, numbness.

— *OBJECTIVE DATA* (observed) —

Nonblanchable erythema, denuded skin, destruction of epidermal and dermal skin layers.

• Compare With

Skin Integrity, Risk for Impaired; Tissue Integrity, Impaired.

Skin Integrity, Risk for Impaired

A state in which a person's skin is at risk of being altered adversely.

• Risk Factors

See related factors for *Impaired Skin Integrity.*

Sleep Pattern Disturbance

Disruption of sleep time that causes discomfort or interferes with desired lifestyle.

• Related Factors

Internal sensory alterations: illness, psychological stress.
External sensory alterations: environmental changes, medication side effects; caregiving responsibilities.

• Defining Characteristics

— *SUBJECTIVE DATA* (reported) —

Difficulty falling asleep, awakening earlier or later than desired, interrupted sleep, not feeling well rested.

— *OBJECTIVE DATA* (observed) —

Changes in behavior and performance (eg, increasing irritability, restlessness, disorientation, lethargy, listlessness), nystagmus, hand tremor, ptosis of eyelid, expressionless face, dark circles under eyes, frequent yawning, changes in posture, thick speech with mispronunciation and incorrect words.

• Compare With

Anxiety; Fatigue.

Social Interaction, Impaired

The state in which a person participates in an insufficient or excessive quantity, or ineffective quality of social exchange.

• Related Factors

Knowledge or skill deficit about ways of enhancing mutuality, communication barriers, self-concept disturbance, absence of available significant others or peers, limited mobility, therapeutic isolation, sociocultural dissonance, environmental barriers, *Altered Thought Processes.*

• Defining Characteristics

— *SUBJECTIVE DATA* (reported) —

Discomfort in social situations; inability to receive or communicate a satisfying sense of belonging, caring, interest, or shared history.

— *OBJECTIVE DATA* (observed) —

Unsuccessful or dysfunctional social interaction behaviors, change in style or pattern of interaction.

• Compare With

Communication, Impaired; Loneliness, Risk for; Social Isolation.

Social Isolation

The state in which a person experiences loneliness and perceives it as a negative or threatened state imposed by others.

• Related Factors

Delay in accomplishing developmental tasks, immature interests, unusual physical appearance, chronic illness, altered mental status, unaccepted social values or behavior, inadequate personal resources, absence of peers, inability to engage in satisfying personal relationships.

• Defining Characteristics

— *SUBJECTIVE DATA* (reported) —

Lack of satisfying personal relationships or significant purpose in life, feelings of rejection or being different from others, inability to meet others' expectations, insecurity in public.

— *OBJECTIVE DATA* (observed) —

Absence of supportive significant other(s); sad, dull affect; communication deficits (eg, language barriers, withdrawal, poor eye contact); hostility in voice or behavior; preoccupation with own thoughts.

• Compare With

Communication, Impaired Verbal; Loneliness, Risk for; Social Interaction, Impaired.

Spiritual Distress

Distress of the human spirit, disruption in the life principle that pervades a person's entire being and integrates and transcends one's biologic and psychosocial nature.

• Related Factors

Separation from religious or cultural ties, challenged belief and value system (eg, due to moral or ethical implications of therapy or intense suffering).

• Defining Characteristics

— *SUBJECTIVE DATA* (reported) —

Concern with meaning of life, death, or belief systems; anger toward God; seeking to understand meaning of suffering, own existence, or moral or ethical implications of therapeutic regimen; inability to participate in usual religious practices; desire to talk with a chaplain or priest; anger toward religious representatives; nightmares, sleep disturbances.

— *OBJECTIVE DATA* (observed) —

Altered behavior or mood (eg, anger, crying, withdrawal, preoccupation, *Anxiety,* hostility, apathy, and so forth), use of gallows humor.

• Compare With

Spiritual Well-Being, Potential for Enhanced.

Spiritual Well-Being, Potential for Enhanced

Spiritual well-being is the process of an individual's developing/unfolding of mystery through harmonious interconnectedness that springs from inner strengths.

• Related Factors

(None listed.)

• Defining Characteristics

— *SUBJECTIVE DATA* (reported) —

A sense of awareness, self-consciousness, sacred source, unifying force, inner core, and transcendence; unfolding mystery; one's experience about life's purpose and meaning, mystery, uncertainty, and struggles; harmonious interconnectedness; relatedness, connectedness, harmony with self, others, higher power/God, and the environment.

• Compare With

Spiritual Distress.

Suffocation, Risk for

The state in which a person is at risk of suffocation (inadequate air available for inhalation).

• Risk Factors

Individual: reduced olfactory sensation or motor abilities, lack of safety education or precautions, cognitive or emotional difficulties, disease or injury process.
Environmental: vehicle warming in closed garage, gas leaks, smoking in bed, use of fuel-burning heaters not vented to outside, clothesline.
Additional factors for children: pillow or propped bottle placed in an infant's crib; playing with plastic bags or balloons, or inserting small objects into mouth or nose; discarded or unused refrigerators or freezers without removed doors; unsupervised bathing or swimming; pacifier hung around neck.

• Compare With

Aspiration, Risk for; Home Maintenance Management, Impaired.

Swallowing, Impaired

The state in which a person has decreased ability to voluntarily pass fluids or solids from the mouth to the stomach.

• Related Factors

Neuromuscular impairment (eg, decreased or absent gag reflex, decreased strength or excursion of muscles involved in mastication or swallowing, perceptual impairment, facial paralysis, postcerebrovascular accident [CVA]); congenital anomalies (cleft palate, tracheoesophageal fistula); mechanical obstruction (eg, edema, tracheostomy tube, tumor); limited awareness; reddened, irritated oropharyngeal cavity; weakness, *Fatigue.*

• Defining Characteristics

— *SUBJECTIVE DATA* (reported) —

Difficulty swallowing.

— *OBJECTIVE DATA* (observed) —

Observed evidence of difficulty in swallowing, stasis or pocketing of food in oral cavity, coughing or choking with swallowing attempts, drooling, evidence of aspiration.

• Compare With

Aspiration, Risk for.

Therapeutic Regimen, Community Management, Ineffective

A pattern of regulating and integrating into community processes programs for treatment of illness and the sequelae of illness that are unsatisfactory for meeting health-related goals.

• Related Factors

(None listed.)

• Defining Characteristics

— *OBJECTIVE DATA* (observed) —

Deficits in persons and programs to be accountable for illness care of aggregates, deficits in advocates for aggregates, deficits in community activities for secondary and tertiary prevention, illness symptoms above the norm expected for the number and type of population, number of health care resources are insufficient for the incidence or prevalence of illness(es), unavailable health care resources for illness care, unexpected acceleration of illness(es).

Therapeutic Regimen: Families, Ineffective Management of

A pattern of regulating and integrating into family processes a program for treatment of illness and the sequelae of illness that is unsatisfactory for meeting specific goals.

• Related Factors

Complexity of health care system, complexity of therapeutic regimen, decisional conflicts, economic difficulties, excessive demands made on individual or family, family conflicts.

• Defining Characteristics

— *SUBJECTIVE DATA* (reported) —

Desire to manage the treatment of illness and prevention of the sequelae, verbalized difficulty with regulation/integration of one or more effects or prevention of complication, verbalizes that family did not take action to reduce risk factors for progression of illness and sequelae.

— *OBJECTIVE DATA* (observed) —

Inappropriate family activities for meeting the goals of a treatment or prevention program, acceleration (expected or unexpected) of illness symptom of a family member, lack of attention to illness and its sequelae.

Therapeutic Regimen: Individual, Effective Management of

A pattern of regulating and integrating into daily living a program for treatment of illness and its sequelae that is satisfactory for meeting specific health goals.

• Related Factors

(None listed.)

• Defining Characteristics

— *SUBJECTIVE DATA* (reported) —

Desire to manage the treatment of illness and prevention of sequelae, verbalized intent to reduce risk factors for progression of illness and sequelae.

— *OBJECTIVE DATA* (observed) —

Appropriate choices of daily activities for meeting the goals of a treatment or prevention program, illness symptoms are within a normal range of expectation.

Management of Therapeutic Regimen, Ineffective Individual

A state in which a person has a pattern of regulating and integrating into daily living a program for treatment of illness (and sequelae) that is unsatisfactory for meeting specific health goals.

• Related Factors

Complexity of health care system or therapeutic regimen, mistrust of regimen or health care personnel, inadequate assistive resources (eg, written schedule to follow regimen, devices to make following regimen easier), economic difficulties, excessive demands on individual or family, family conflict or patterns of health care inconsistent with therapeutic regimen, social support deficits.

• Defining Characteristics

— *SUBJECTIVE DATA* (reported) —

Desire to manage the illness and prevent sequelae; difficulty with regulation or integration of prescribed regimens for treatment of illness and its effects, or prevention of complications; report that no actions are being taken to include treatment regimens in daily routines or to reduce risk factors for progression of illness and sequelae.

— *OBJECTIVE DATA* (observed) —

Acceleration or lack of improvement of symptoms, choices of daily living ineffective for meeting the goals of treatment or prevention program.

• Compare With

Decisional Conflict; Health Maintenance, Altered; Home Maintenance Management, Impaired; Knowledge Deficit; Powerlessness.

Thermoregulation, Ineffective

The state in which a person's temperature fluctuates between hypothermia and hyperthermia.

• Related Factors

Trauma, illness, immaturity, aging, fluctuating environmental temperature.

• Defining Characteristics

— *OBJECTIVE DATA* (observed) —

Fluctuations in body temperature above or below the normal range.

• Compare With

Body Temperature, Risk for Altered.

Thought Processes, Altered

The state in which a person experiences a disruption in such mental activities as conscious thought, reality orientation, problem solving, judgment, and comprehension. (Adapted from Carpenito, 1997a)

• Related Factors

Medications, substance abuse, electrolyte imbalance, depression, dementia, bipolar disorders, borderline personality, multiple demands or stressors, sleep deprivation, sensory bombardment.

• Defining Characteristics

— *SUBJECTIVE DATA* (reported) —

Inaccurate interpretation of internal or external stimuli, hallucinations, delusions, phobias, obsessions, *Anxiety, Fear.*

— *OBJECTIVE DATA* (observed) —

Distractibility, cognitive dissonance, memory deficit, egocentricity, hyper- or hypovigilance, confusion, disorientation.

• Compare With

Sensory–Perceptual Alterations.

Tissue Integrity, Impaired

A state in which a person experiences damage to mucous membrane, corneal, integumentary, or subcutaneous tissue.

• Related Factors

Altered circulation, nutritional deficit or excess, fluid deficit or excess, *Knowledge Deficit,* impaired mobility, chemical irritants (body secretions or excretions, medications), temperature extremes, mechanical factors (pressure, shear, friction), radiation.

• Defining Characteristics

— *SUBJECTIVE DATA* (reported) —

Pain.

— *OBJECTIVE DATA* (observed) —

Damaged or destroyed tissue (corneal, mucous membrane, integumentary, or subcutaneous).

• Compare With

Oral Mucous Membrane, Altered; Skin Integrity, Impaired.

Tissue Perfusion, Altered (Specify: renal, cerebral, cardiopulmonary, GI, peripheral)

The state in which a person experiences a decrease in nutrition and oxygenation at the cellular level because of deficit in capillary blood supply.

• Related Factors

Interruption of arterial or venous flow, exchange problems, hypovolemia, hypervolemia, pathology.

• Defining Characteristics

— *SUBJECTIVE DATA* (reported) —

Pain, claudication.

— *OBJECTIVE DATA* (observed) —

Cold skin temperature, poor peripheral pulse quality, blue-black, pale skin, slow healing of lesions.

• Author's Note

The defining characteristics listed relate to altered peripheral tissue perfusion; the other subcomponents haven't been developed.

• Compare With

Activity Intolerance; Peripheral Neurovascular Dysfunction, Risk for.

Trauma, Risk for

The state in which a person is at risk of injury to tissues (eg, wound, burn, fracture).

• Risk Factors

Individual: weakness; vision, balance, cognitive, or emotional difficulties; reduced temperature or tactile sensation; reduced hand–eye coordination, or large or small muscle coordination; lack of safety education or precautions; insufficient finances to purchase safety equipment or effect repairs; history of previous trauma.

Environmental: slippery floors, stairs, or walkways (highly waxed, wet spots, icy or snowy spots); unanchored rugs or electrical wires; bathtub without hand grip or antislip equipment; unsteady ladders or chairs; unlighted rooms; unsturdy or absent stair rails; obstructed passageways; inappropriate call-for-aid mechanisms for immobile individuals; potential for igniting gas leaks; delayed lighting of gas burner or oven; experimenting with chemical or gasoline; unscreened fires or heaters; wearing plastic apron or flowing clothes around open flame; inadequately stored combustibles or corrosives (matches, oily rags, lye); overloaded fuse boxes; contact with rapidly moving machinery, industrial belts, or pulleys; sliding on coarse bed linen; struggling within restraints; faulty electrical plugs, frayed wires, or defective appliances; contact with acids or alkalis; playing with fireworks or gunpowder; contact with intense cold; overexposure to sun, sun lamps; cracked dishware or glasses; knives stored uncovered; guns or ammunition stored unlocked; large icicles hanging from roof; exposure to dangerous machinery; high crime neighborhood and vulnerable clients; driving a mechanically unsafe vehicle, after partaking in alcohol or drugs, at excessive speeds, or without necessary visual or hearing aids; smoking in bed or near oxygen; overloaded electrical outlets; grease waste collected on stoves; thin or worn potholders; misuse of bicycle or motorcycle helmets; unsafe road or road-crossing conditions; play or work near vehicle pathways (eg, driveways, lanes, railroad tracks).

Additional for children: unsafe storage of medications or potential poisons; inadequate stair gates; unsafe window protection; appliance cords or pot handles within reach; unsupervised bathing, swimming, or play; flammable toys or clothing; toys with sharp edges or small parts that can be removed; toys not approved for ages of children in home; balloons; availability of matches, candles, and cigarettes; inadequate car seats; absence of bicycle wheel guard or helmet for child riding on back; absence of adequate fences or gates in pool area; unfamiliar pets (dogs, cats).

• Compare With

Injury, Risk for.

Unilateral Neglect

The state in which a person is unaware of the hemiplegic side of his or her body, or unaware of objects, persons, or sounds on the hemiplegic side of the body.

• Related Factors

Effects of stroke, brain tumor, or brain injury (hemianopsia, one-sided blindness, perceptual disturbances).

• Defining Characteristics

— *OBJECTIVE DATA* (observed) —

Failure to see, hear, or feel stimuli on affected side; failure to purposefully use extremities on affected side; lack of awareness of positioning of extremities on affected side.

• Compare With

Sensory–Perceptual Alterations, Visual; Self-Care Deficit.

Urinary Elimination, Altered

The state in which a person experiences a disturbance in urine elimination.

• Related Factors

Many causes, including problems with urinary tract structure or function, urinary tract infection, neurogenic disorders, side effects of medications.

• Defining Characteristics

— *SUBJECTIVE DATA* (reported) —

Dysuria, urgency, frequency, hesitancy, incontinence, nocturia.

— *OBJECTIVE DATA* (observed) —

Residual urine volumes greater than 100 mL, incontinence, enuresis.

• Clinical Alert

Report prolonged *Altered Urinary Elimination* (may be a sign of medical diagnoses such as *diabetes, infection, enlarged prostate,* and *cancer*).

• Compare With

Urinary Incontinence, Functional; Urinary Incontinence, Reflex; Urinary Incontinence, Stress; Urinary Incontinence, Total; Urinary Incontinence, Urge; Urinary Retention.

Urinary Incontinence, Functional

The state in which a person experiences an involuntary, unpredictable passage of urine.

• Related Factors

Altered environment; sensory, cognitive, or mobility deficits; medication side effects; neurogenic disorders; loss of perineal muscle tone; decreased bladder capacity.

• Defining Characteristics

— *SUBJECTIVE DATA* (reported) —

Urge to void strong enough to result in loss of urine before reaching bedpan or commode.

— *OBJECTIVE DATA* (observed) —

Episodic involuntary urination.

• Compare With

Urinary Elimination, Altered; Urinary Incontinence, Reflex; Urinary Incontinence, Stress; Urinary Incontinence, Total; Urinary Incontinence, Urge.

Urinary Incontinence, Reflex

The state in which a person experiences an involuntary loss of urine, occurring at somewhat predictable intervals when a specific bladder volume is reached.

• Related Factors

Neurologic impairment (eg, spinal cord lesion that interferes with conduction of cerebral messages above the level of the reflex arc).

• Defining Characteristics

— *SUBJECTIVE DATA* (reported) —

No awareness of bladder filling, no urge to void or feelings of bladder fullness.

— *OBJECTIVE DATA* (observed) —

Involuntary urination at somewhat predictable intervals.

• Compare With

Urinary Elimination, Altered; Urinary Incontinence, Functional; Urinary Incontinence, Stress; Urinary Incontinence, Total; Urinary Incontinence, Urge.

Urinary Incontinence, Stress

The state in which a person experiences a loss of urine occurring with increased abdominal pressure.

• Related Factors

Degenerative changes or weakness in pelvic muscles and structural supports, high intra-abdominal pressure (eg, obesity, gravid uterus, coughing), incompetent bladder outlet, overdistention between voidings.

• Defining Characteristics

— *SUBJECTIVE DATA* (reported) —

Urinary urgency; urinary incontinence with coughing, sneezing.

— *OBJECTIVE DATA* (observed) —

Dribbling with increased abdominal pressure, urinary frequency (more often than every 2 hours).

• Compare With

Urinary Elimination, Altered; Urinary Incontinence, Functional; Urinary Incontinence, Reflex; Urinary Incontinence, Total; Urinary Incontinence, Urge; Urinary Retention.

Urinary Incontinence, Total

The state in which a person experiences a continuous and unpredictable loss of urine.

• Related Factors

Neuropathy preventing transmission of reflex indicating bladder fullness, neurologic dysfunction causing triggering of micturition at unpredictable times, independent contraction of detrusor reflex due to surgery, trauma or disease affecting spinal cord nerves, anomaly (fistula).

• Defining Characteristics

— *SUBJECTIVE DATA* (reported) —

Unawareness of bladder filling or incontinence, decreased sensation of perineal area.

— *OBJECTIVE DATA* (observed) —

Constant flow of urine at unpredictable times without urinary distention, incontinence not responding to treatment.

• Compare With

Urinary Incontinence, Functional; Urinary Incontinence, Reflex; Urinary Incontinence, Stress; Urinary Incontinence, Urge.

Urinary Incontinence, Urge

The state in which a person experiences involuntary passage of urine occurring soon after a strong sense of urgency to void.

• Related Factors

Decreased bladder capacity (eg, history of PID, abdominal surgeries, indwelling urinary catheter), irritation of bladder stretch receptors causing spasm (eg, bladder infection), alcohol, caffeine, increased fluids, increased urine concentration, overdistention of bladder, enlarged prostate.

• Defining Characteristics

— *SUBJECTIVE DATA* (reported) —

Urgency, inability to reach bedpan or commode in time, frequent voiding.

— *OBJECTIVE DATA* (observed) —

Frequent urination, voiding immediately after urge to urinate.

• Compare With

Urinary Elimination, Altered; Urinary Incontinence, Functional; Urinary Incontinence, Reflex; Urinary Incontinence, Stress; Urinary Incontinence, Total; Urinary Retention.

Urinary Retention

The state in which a person experiences incomplete emptying of the bladder.

• Related Factors

High urethral pressure caused by weak detrusor muscles, inhibition of reflex arc, strong sphincter, blockage, medication side effects.

• Defining Characteristics

— *SUBJECTIVE DATA* (reported) —

Sensation of bladder fullness, dysuria.

— *OBJECTIVE DATA* (observed) —

Bladder distention; urine loss or voiding in small, frequent amounts; absence of urine output; dribbling; residual urine $>$100 mL.

• Compare With

Urinary Elimination, Altered; Urinary Incontinence, Stress; Urinary Incontinence, Urge.

Ventilation, Inability to Sustain Spontaneous

A state in which the response pattern of decreased energy reserves results in a person's inability to maintain breathing adequate to support life.

• Related Factors

Metabolic factors, respiratory muscle fatigue.

• Defining Characteristics

— *SUBJECTIVE DATA* (reported) —

Dyspnea, apprehension.

— *OBJECTIVE DATA* (observed) —

Bradypnea, tachypnea, increased restlessness, decreased cooperation, increased use of accessory muscles, decreased tidal volume, increased heart rate, decreased Po_2, increased PCo_2, decreased oxygen saturation.

• Clinical Alert

These defining characteristics describe a degree of respiratory distress which is life-threatening and requires immediate initiation of physician-prescribed interventions.

• Compare With

Ventilatory Weaning Response, Dysfunctional.

Ventilatory Weaning Response, Dysfunctional (DVWR)

The state in which someone cannot adjust to lowered levels of mechanical ventilator support, which interrupts and prolongs the weaning process.

• Related Factors

Excessive airway secretions, sleep deprivation, inadequate nutrition, pain or discomfort, lack of trust in caregivers, insufficient information related to weaning process, perceived need for ventilator, prolonged ventilator dependence, previous unsuccessful weaning attempts, lack of motivation, nonsupportive environment, inappropriate pacing of weaning plan, *Fatigue, Anxiety, Fear.*

• Defining Characteristics

— *SUBJECTIVE DATA* (reported) —

During weaning periods: increased need for oxygen, breathing discomfort, fatigue, warmth; increased concentration on breathing; apprehension.

— *OBJECTIVE DATA* (observed) —

During weaning periods: restlessness; increased blood pressure, heart rate, and respiratory rate; hypervigilance; lack of response to coaching; diaphoresis; wide-eyed look; decreased breath sounds; pallor, cyanosis; use of accessory muscles for respiration; agitation; deterioration in arterial blood gases or oxygen saturation; shallow, gasping breaths; paradoxical abdominal breathing; decreased consciousness level.

Violence, Risk for: Self-Directed or Directed at Others

A state in which a person demonstrates behaviors that can be physically harmful either to the self or others.

• Related Factors

Antisocial character; history of aggressive acts; child or spouse abuse; organic brain syndrome; temporal lobe epilepsy; toxic reactions to medications, alcohol, illegal drugs; catatonic or manic excitement; panic states; hallucinations; rage reactions; suicidal behavior.

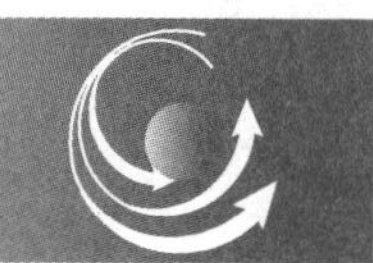

Example Responses to Practice Sessions

PRACTICE SESSION I

1. a. *Assessment* involves examining and interviewing the patient to determine health status. During *Diagnosis*, you analyze patient information and identify the problems requiring nursing or medical treatment. In *Planning*, the expected outcomes—goals of care—are determined, and the treatment plan is developed and recorded. In *Implementation*, you put the plan into action. Finally, In *Evaluation*, you evaluate whether the patient achieved the expected outcomes, or goals, and modify or terminate the plan as indicated. b. Paraphrase any of the benefits listed in Display 1–2. **2.** Use of nursing process is a requirement set forth by national practice standards (see Display 1–1); it provides the basis for questions on state board exams; it promotes critical thinking in the clinical setting. **3.** The problems identified in *Diagnosis* are based on the information collected during *Assessment*. The outcomes identified during *Planning* are based on the problems determined in *Diagnosis*. The interventions used in *Implementation* are based on the outcomes identified during *Planning*.

PRACTICE SESSION II

1. You can decide this by comparing yourself with Display 1–6. **3.** Compare your answer with Display 1–5. **4.** See Display 1–8.

PRACTICE SESSION III

Part I. 1. a. Tell me how you're feeling. b. How was your dinner? c. How do you feel about being here? d. Describe what you're feeling; tell me how you're feeling. **2.** a. So, you've been sick off and on for a month. What do you mean by *sick off and on*? b. You feel like nothing ever goes right for you. What's been happening? c. You have a pain in your side that comes and goes—can you explain more? d. You've had a funny feeling for a week. What do you mean by *funny*? **3.** a) C b) E c) S d) L e) O f) C g) S h) L i) O j) L k) E. **4.** d. How do you feel about feeding Susan? h. How would it be if your family visited? j. How do you feel about practicing more?

Part II. 1. a. You have a lot of ground-in dirt here. What's it from? b. I feel a lump on the back of your head. How did it happen? Does it hurt when I touch it? c. Your breathing is a little fast. How do you feel? d. Your eye seems inflamed. How does it feel? e. I see you have some cavities. When did you see a dentist last? **2.** a. Show me where (and examine that area). Is there anything you think causes it? b. Show me where (and examine that area). Tell me more about how it feels. c. That's a common symptom of infection. Let's get a urine sample (and examine it). d. Where do you feel this bloating? Your stomach? Ankles? Where? (and examine the area).

PRACTICE SESSION IV

Part I. **1.** 51 years old, no pain, feels better, feels relieved, denies being weary. **2.** Lab study results, talking slowly, frequent sighing, vital signs.
Part II. a. All the data listed under Part I, numbers 1 and 2. b. Physical condition seems to be improving. He is more comfortable. Seems weary/tired.
Part III. **1.** Certainly valid: Lab studies, talking slowly, frequent sighing. Probably valid: 51 years old, no pain, feels better, vital signs. Possibly valid: Weary/tired. **2.** Compare age with birth date. Ask probing questions to clarify comfort state (*Are you sure you don't have any discomfort*?) Look for nonverbal signs of discomfort (eg, rubbing hand on chest). Spend quality time with him discussing how he feels physically and psychologically. Recheck vital signs.

PRACTICE SESSION V

1. You need to do both to facilitate recognition of both possible nursing problems and medical problems (see page 59). **2.** *Body systems:* Resp: 5, 6, 8, 10, 13, 14. Card: 6. Circ: 6, 15. GI: 9. Neuro: none specifically listed GU: none listed, although you might have chosen to put 11 (childbirth) here. Skin: None listed. *Holistic nursing model:* (this organizes data according to Functional Health Patterns, but you may have chosen another model) Nutritional–Metabolic: 5, 6, 9, 10, 11, 13, 14, 15. Elimination: None listed. Activity-Exercise: 3, 8. Cognitive-perceptual: None listed. Sleep-rest: 8. Self-perception–self-concept: Role-relationship: 2, 3, 7. Sexual–reproductive: 1, 2. Coping-Stress: 10, 12. Value–belief: 4. 3. You should think how you can gain the missing information.

PRACTICE SESSION VI

1. a) N b) A c) N d) A e) A f) N g) A h) A i) N j) A. **2.** Ask Mr. Moran to describe his daily activities. Ask him whether he has assistance with these routines. Ask what would make following the routines easier, how he could be more independent. Ask him to tell you any specific problems he sees in accomplishing daily routines. **3.** Ask Mr. Moran about his smoking history. If he's smoked, determine whether he still smokes. Ask Mr. Moran about his environment at home (air quality, such as humidity or dryness). Find out if he's ever been tested for allergies and whether contact with potential allergens has been avoided. Ask Mr. Moran to name three things that aggravate his breathing problems and three things that might help him do better.

PRACTICE SESSION VII

1. a. You may perform an action if you're qualified to do so (if you've demonstrated competency and have been given the authority). **b.** See Table 3–2. **2.** 1) t 2) g 3) b 4) a 5) h 6) d 7) l 8) p 9) m 10) n 11) r 12) o 13) e 14) k 15) f 16) s 17) c 18) q 19) i 20) j 21) u. **3. a.** 1) C 2) N 3) C 4) N 5) C 6) N **b.** 1) C 2) N 3) N 4) C 5) N 6) N 7) C 8) C 9) N 10) C 11) N 12) N 13) C 14) C **4.** Both models focus on treating health problems. The PPM model has a stronger focus on *early intervention* to prevent or manage potential complications.

PRACTICE SESSION VIII

1) b 2) a 3) c 4) e 5) g 6) h 7) f 8) d.

PRACTICE SESSION IX

Part I. 1. a. Problem: Urge incontinence. Cause: inability to hold large amounts of urine. Signs and symptoms: voiding immediately upon realization of need to void. b. Problem: Anticipatory Grieving. Cause: related to impending death of mother. Signs and symptoms: statements of extreme sadness over impending death. **2.** Because if they had signs and symptoms, they'd be *actual* diagnoses.
Part II. 1. *Ineffective Airway Clearance related to copious secretions as evidenced by inability to clear tracheostomy without suction.* **2.** *Altered Nutrition: Less than Body Requirements related to poor appetite as evidenced by 15 lb below recommended weight.* **3.** *Powerlessness related to quadriplegia and rigorous physical therapy schedule as evidenced by report of depression and feelings of having no choices.*
Part III. 1. *Possible Ineffective Individual Coping.* **2.** *Risk for Fluid Volume Deficit related to fever.* **3.** *Risk for Ineffective Airway Clearance related to smoking history and recent general anesthesia.* **4.** *Possible Sexual Dysfunction.*
Part IV. A. 1, **4**, **7**, & **9** are correct. **B. 2.** May be legally incriminating. **3.** Addresses two problems in one diagnosis, isn't specific about where the pain is, isn't specific about what about the surgery is causing anxiety (eg, knowing too little? knowing too much?). **5.** Makes a value judgment that someone who's an atheist has *Spiritual Distress* **6.** Doesn't focus on the *response* to the mastectomy or cancer. **8.** Renames a medical problem to make it sound like a nursing diagnosis. **10.** Neither the problem nor the related factors can be treated by nurse-prescribed interventions.

PRACTICE SESSION X

Part I. 1. PC: thrombus formation, phlebitis, extravasation, fluid overload related to IV. **2.** PC: brain swelling, bleeding,, increased intracranial pressure related to concussion. **3.** PC: arrhythmias, hypotension, shock, congestive heart failure, pulmonary edema, reinfarction, embolus, cerebrovascular accident, cardiac arrest related to MI. **4.** PC: electrolyte imbalance, abdominal distention, bleeding, misplacement of the tube related to nasogastric tube. PC: abdominal distention related to disease process.
Part II. You would ask a question like, *Looking at the big picture of this patient's situation, is it likely that he/she will be able to reach the desired outcomes in the expected timeframe using only nursing expertise for planning and management of care*? See *Identifying the Need for Multidisciplinary Approaches* on page 106.

PRACTICE SESSION XI

Strengths: normal vital signs, moves all extremities with equal strength, strong peripheral pulses, abdomen soft, equal pupils.
Nursing Diagnoses: *Risk for Injury related to dizziness: Risk for Altered Patterns of Urinary Elimination related to inability to use the bed pan: Fear related to hospitalization as evidenced by statements of fear of hospitals and needles. Possible Altered Family Processes.*

Collaborative Problems: PC: increased intracranial pressure, bleeding, phlebitis or extravasation at intravenous site.

PRACTICE SESSION XII

1. Promoting communication, directing care and documentation, providing a record that can be used for evaluation and research, providing insurance companies with a record of care requirements. **2.** Problems (eg, *Self-Care Deficit: Dressing*): outcomes (eg, will be able to dress self completely by discharge); interventions (eg, have client practice buttoning clothing three times a day). **3.** Patient's perception of priorities, understanding of the whole picture of problems, patient's prognosis and overall health status, expected length of stay or contact, presence of clinical guidelines or critical paths related to specific situation. **4.** Severe dyspnea. Severe breathing problems are top priority unless the patient is hemorrhaging. **5.** Your state practice act, ANA standards, specialty organization standards (if you're in a specialty unit, like maternity), JCAHO standards, unique standards of the facility where you're working. **6.** Knowing the overall discharge outcomes helps you decide which problems need to be given a high priority in order to be ready for discharge in a timely fashion.

PRACTICE SESSION XIII

Part I. 1. Outcomes are used to direct interventions, motivate patients and care givers, and evaluate progress. **2.** Outcome, goal, objective. **3.** Outcome. **4.** a. Report the problem to whomever is responsible for achieving the outcome. b. Develop and initiate a plan of care to treat the problem. **5.** All nurses are responsible for detecting and reporting patients who may require case management (ie, patients who may require extra resources to achieve the expected outcomes in a timely manner).
Part II. 1. Measurable verbs help everyone to stay focused on observable data that will let you know how well the patient is progressing toward outcome achievement. For examples of measurable verbs, see page 122. **2.** Subject: Who is the person expected to achieve the goal? Verb: What actions must the person take to achieve the goal? Condition: Under what circumstances is the person to perform the actions? Performance Criteria: How well is the person to perform the actions? Target Time: By when is the person expected to be able to perform the actions? **3.** The following are incorrect. a. The verb isn't measurable. c. Nonspecific. How will we measure what is meant by "will improve"? f. No time frame listed; verb isn't measurable and observable. i. Verb isn't measurable. **4.** a. After increasing roughage intake, Miss Pierce will report having one soft, formed, bowel movement every 1 to 2 days beginning Thursday. b. After Dianne begins performing daily tooth brushing, flossing, and gum care, her gums will be pink and healthy looking (by 10/28). c. The skin around Mr. Culp's incision will be clean without signs of redness or irritation. d. After instructions, Mrs. Sovosky will correctly express needs by using flash cards (by 4/26). e. After a visit by the chaplain, Heidi will relate feeling more at peace, as evidenced by reporting that the chaplain reinforced that it's okay to miss Mass when you're ill. f. Miss O'Dell will demonstrate how to feed herself with the use of padded spoons by 5/9. 4. a. Will demonstrate healthy looking gums, without redness or irritation by Jan 15. b. Will not demonstrate signs and symptoms of Impaired Skin Integrity in the rectal area and area will be kept clean. c. Will be able to communicate basic needs through use of flash cards and through an interpreter when required.
Part III. a) C, P b) A c) C d) C, P
Part IV. a. View film on infant nutrition and formula feedings on 4/5. Describes the steps involved in sterilizing formula on 4/5. Demonstrate sterilizing baby formula on 4/6. b. Discuss with primary nurse on 2/2 how patient feels about going home. c. Attend group diabetic class on nutrition on 10/11. Discuss with primary nurse the relationship between blood sugar

levels and eating certain foods on 10/11. Review printed diet restrictions on 10/11. d. Attend group diabetic class on insulin administration and monitoring of blood sugar level on 7/29. View teaching film on insulin administration and monitoring of blood sugar level on 7/29. Observe the nurse demonstrating the correct procedures for insulin administration and for testing blood sugar level on 7/30. Practice insulin self-administration based on morning blood sugar readings beginning 7/31.

PRACTICE SESSION XIV

Part I. 1. Classifying interventions into direct and indirect interventions allows you to examine nursing activities and time spent in direct contact with patients and activities and time spent performing activities on behalf of the patient, but away from the patient (eg, analyzing lab studies). **2.** See = What must be *assessed or observed* related to the intervention; do = what must be *done*; teach = what must be *taught or reinforced*; record = what must be *recorded* related to the intervention. **3.** What can be done about the cause(s) of this problem? What can be done to help this specific person achieve this specific outcome? **4.** See Display 4–7.
Part II. 1. Monitor skin integrity, especially over bony prominences, with each position change. Post at bedside a schedule for turning every 2 hours, enlisting the client's maximum participation. Keep an air mattress on the bed. Ensure adequate vitamin C and protein intake. Keep sheets clean, dry, and unwrinkled. **2.** *Preoperatively:* Determine patient and family knowledge of coughing and deep breathing with incisional splinting. Teach as indicated and have patient return demonstration. *Postoperatively*: Monitor for incisional pain and medicate pm before pain is too intense. Teach the importance of asking for pain medication before pain is severe, changing positions, ambulating early and coughing and deep breathing. Record pain level after medication is given. Record breath sounds q4h. Help client to cough and deep breath q2h the day of surgery and first postoperative day. **3.** Monitor daily bowel movements. Teach the relationship between exercise, diet, fluid intake, and bowel elimination. Develop a plan to increase roughage and fluid intake, and to increase exercise gradually (eg, using stairs instead of elevator).
Part III. 1. PC: Extravasation, phlebitis, thrombus formation, fluid overload, infection. Plan: Follow hospital policies or standards for care of IV therapy. Monitor vital signs q4h. Monitor IV site for signs and symptoms of infection, extravasation, phlebitis, thrombus q4h. Instruct patient to report discomfort or swelling at IV site. **2.** PC: Hypoglycemia/hyperglycemia. Plan: Follow hospital policies or standards for care of diabetics. Record daily caloric intake. Record blood sugars q4h. Instruct patient to report symptoms of dizziness or "feeling funny" in any way. **3.** PC: Infection, blockage of the catheter, bleeding. Plan: Follow hospital policies and standards for Foley catheter care. Monitor temperature q4–8h. Monitor urine color, odor, and amount. Record intake and output q8h. Monitor meatus for drainage or bleeding. Instruct patient to report catheter or bladder discomfort.

PRACTICE SESSION XV

1. a. Even though the woman is young and has had routine surgery, I wouldn't delegate the task. b. Because it's the first time she's getting out of bed and you don't really know how she will respond. (See *When Should You Delegate*? on page 158. **2.** a. The nurse is accountable because she knew the UAP was leaving the child in the care of his mother, who may not have been aware of the possibility of her child sneaking out while she was in the bathroom. b. The nurse could have assigned another UAP to monitor the child or she could have clearly cautioned the mother not to leave her child unattended for any reason (rather, the mother should call if she needed to go to the bathroom or whatever). **3.** a) You perform a complete assessment and determine whether the patient is progressing as expected according to plan of care. For example, if the plan includes a critical path that states "chest tubes will be out by the second postoperative day," and the patient still has chest tubes, you've identified a variance in care, b) You should perform additional assessment to determine whether the delay is justified or whether actions need to be taken to improve the patient's likelihood of achieving the outcome. c) Additional assessments and interventions that may be required for the patient to progress may be omitted, resulting in harm to the patient or delays in recovery. d) If the patient is harmed, you may be accused of negligence. If there are delays in recovery, you may be accused of giving substandard care.

PRACTICE SESSION XVI

1. Patient records: 1. Communicate care to other health care professionals who need to be able to find out what you've done and how the patient's doing. 2. Help identify patterns of responses and changes in status. 3. Provide a foundation for evaluation, research, and improvement of the quality of care. 4. Create a legal document that may later be used in court to evaluate the type of care rendered. Your records can be your best friend or worst enemy—the best defense that you actually observed or did something is the fact that you made a note of it. 5. Supply validation for insurance purposes. The saying goes, "If it's not documented, they won't pay." **2.** You'll be more accurate when the information is fresh in your mind. Charting what you've done often jogs your mind to recognize when you've forgotten to do something *else* you should have done. **3. DAR:** D—States she feels like she's choking, but is afraid to cough because of incisional pain. A—Assisted to splint with pillow. R—Coughed up gray mucous plug. **DIE:** D—States she feels like she's choking, but is afraid to cough because of incisional pain. I—Assisted to splint incision with a pillow. E—Coughed up gray mucus plug. Lungs clear. **AIR-A:** A—States she feels like she's choking, but is afraid to cough because of incisional pain. I—Assisted to splint incision with a pillow. R—Coughed up gray mucus plug. Lungs clear. A—Emphasized importance of reporting pain that interferes with breathing. **4.** a. It's judgmental and has no supporting evidence. b. It has no supporting evidence—states opinion, not facts. **5.** You should have drawn a line through the note, then written the word *error*, followed by your initials.

PRACTICE SESSION XVII

Part I. 1) P 2) A 3) N. Insulin demand is affected by increased exercise. 4) P. 5) P. Fever and heat are also signs of infection.
Part II. Continue the plan if the patient hasn't achieved outcomes, but you haven't identified any factors that impeded or enhanced care. **Modify the plan** when outcomes haven't been achieved, and you've identified factors that enhanced or impeded care. **Terminate the plan** if the patient has achieved outcomes and demonstrates ability to care for himself.

PRACTICE SESSION XVIII

1. Information gained from these studies improves the quality and efficiency of patient care, and helps identify ways of improving nurses' job satisfaction. **2.** Considering all three types of evaluation—outcome (results), process (method), and structure (setting)—provides a comprehensive examination of care management. **3.** The terms all basically mean the same thing (see Display 6–3). **4.** Staff nurses have three main responsibilities: 1) Reporting areas that could be improved to their supervisor. 2) Keeping accurate records. 3) Applying results of QI studies to their practice.

APPENDIX A

American Nurses Association Code for Nurses†

As a nurse, you must:

✓ **Provide** services with respect for human dignity and the uniqueness of the client, unrestricted by considerations of social or economic status, personal attributes, or the nature of health problems.

✓ **Safeguard** the:
- client's right to privacy by judiciously protecting information of a confidential nature.
- client and public when health care and safety are affected by the incompetent, unethical, or illegal practice of any person.

✓ **Assume** responsibility and accountability for individual nursing judgments and actions.

✓ **Maintain** competence in nursing.

✓ **Exercise** informed judgment and use individual competence and qualifications as criteria in seeking consultation, accepting responsibilities, and delegating nursing activities to others.

✓ **Participate** in the profession's:
- activities that contribute to the ongoing development of the profession's body of knowledge.
- efforts to implement and improve standards of nursing.
- efforts to establish and maintain conditions of employment conducive to high-quality nursing care.
- efforts to protect the public from misinformation and misrepresentation and to maintain the integrity of nursing.

✓ **Collaborate** with members of the health care professions and other citizens in promoting community and national efforts to meet the health needs of the public.

---

†Adapted from *Code for Nurses With Interpretive Statements* (ANA, 1985).

APPENDIX

B Sample Critical Path and Care Map™*

*Adapted with permission from the Center for Case Management, South Natick, MA.

Brighton Medical Center Case CareMap™
Profile: Uncomplicated MI

Case Manager:__________

(Addressograph)

Patient Problem/ Nursing Diagnosis	DAY 1	DAY 2	DAY 3	DAY 4	DAY 5	DAY 6
Pain R/T ischemia	Pt. will verbalize pain or discomfort appropriately to RN	Pt will be pain free	—	—	—	Pt. will be pain free at discharge
Activity intolerance R/T ischemia	Pt. will be able to tolerate BSC without chest pain Pt. can participate in "PT protocol" without chest pain	Pt. can participate in "PT protocol" without chest pain	—	—	—	Pt will be discharged at anticipated activity tolerance as evidenced by B/P does not change by 20 torr and HR does not change by 20 BPM
Knowledge deficit R/T new MI	Pt. can state why admitted to hospital Pt. will understand the importance of notifying RN of chest pain	Pt. will demonstrate a readiness to learn Pt. will begin to read MI packet	Pt. will be able to state what an MI and angina are and risk factors & use of sublingual nitrates	Pt. demonstrates understanding of diet by making appropriate choices on menu Pt. can verbalize discharge needs	Pt. can verbalize community resources Pt. can take own pulse	Pt. can verbalize activity restrictions and rationale. Pt. can restate discharge instructions. Pt. will have completed all MI teaching packet goals
Anxiety R/T hospitalization	Pt. can verbalize fears and concerns related to hospitalization	—	Pt. displays appropriate coping skills	—	—	Pt. can identify appropriate resources and support systems
Potential for injury R/T bleeding (TPA)	Pt. will verbalize understanding of reasons to notify RN of signs of bleeding	—	—	—	—	Pt. can state rationale for risk factors of anticoagulation therapy

Critical Path						
Consults	Notify ER attending & family physician, Social Services, Quality Review, Case Manager	PT Dietary consultation	Social Services • home care referral	• Pharmacy consult (coumadin teaching)		
Tests	MCPs q 8° × 3 EKG, routine lab work/coag. CXR. O_2 sat	EKG • MCP • 2 D echo • routine labs • O_2 sat	• EKG • schedule Holter monitor	Holter monitor	• coag. • routine labs • schedule stress test	• stress test
Treatments	I & O, weight, IV access, cardiac monitoring. B/P, V/S monitoring	• weight — Same as Day 1	D/C cardiac monitoring & transfer	IV access — Same as Day 3	IV access	D/C IV
Meds	• O_2 • Pa • Ntg • Reg meds • Lidocaine • MS • Sleeper Heparin • Tylenol • Beta Blockers • Ca channel blockers and anxiety agent Stool Softener	Same • wean Lido • wean Ntg • O_2	Same wean Lido wean Ntg	Same Assess anticoag therapy (D/C heparin & consider ASA)		Discharge prescription with completed discharge form
Diet	Cardiac Diet	—	—	—	—	—
Activity	Bedrest with BSC ADL protocol	PT protocol — —	— — —	— — —	— — —	— — —
Teaching	Orientation to unit & routine Dietary reading material	MI packet progressive dietary teaching	—	Evaluate process & target problem areas • Coumadin teaching info bracelet	—	Discharge instruction review
Discharge Planning		Share CareMap if appropriate	Update to Social Service from QR transfer to general floor	As per Social Service	Consider outpatient needs	Discharge

APPENDIX

C Nursing Interventions Classification (NIC)* Intervention Labels and Codes

Abuse Protection
Abuse Protection: Child
Abuse Protection: Elder
Acid–Base Management
Acid–Base Management Metabolic Acidosis
Acid–Base Management Metabolic Alkalosis
Acid–Base Management Respiratory Acidosis
Acid–Base Management Respiratory Alkalosis
Acid–Base Monitoring
Active Listening
Activity Therapy
Acupressure
Admission Care
Airway Insertion and Stabilization
Airway Management
Airway Suctioning
Allergy Management
Amnioinfusion
Amputation Care
Analgesic Administration
Analgesic Administration: Intraspinal
Anesthesia Administration
Anger Control Assistance
Animal Assisted Therapy
Anticipatory Guidance
Anxiety Reduction
Area Restriction
Art Therapy
Artificial Airway Management
Aspiration Precautions
Assertiveness Training
Attachment Promotion
Autogenic Training
Autotransfusion

Bathing
Bed Rest Care
Bedside Laboratory Testing
Behavior Management
Behavior Management Overactivity/Inattention
Behavior Management Self Harm
Behavior Management Sexual
Behavior Modification
Behavior Modification: Social Skills
Bibliotherapy
Biofeedback
Birthing
Bladder Irrigation
Bleeding Precautions
Bleeding Reduction
Bleeding Reduction: Antepartum Uterus
Bleeding Reduction: Gastrointestinal
Bleeding Reduction: Nasal
Bleeding Reduction: Postpartum Uterus
Bleeding Reduction: Wound
Blood Products Administration
Body Image Enhancement
Body Mechanics Promotion
Bottle Feeding
Bowel Incontinence Care
Bowel Incontinence Care: Encopresis
Bowel Irrigation
Bowel Management
Bowel Training
Breastfeeding Assistance

Calming Technique
Cardiac Care
Cardiac Care: Acute
Cardiac Care: Rehabilitative
Cardiac Precautions
Caregiver Support
Cast Care: Maintenance
Cast Care: Wet
Cerebral Edema Management
Cerebral Perfusion Promotion
Cesarean Section Care
Chemotherapy Management
Chest Physiotherapy
Childbirth Preparation
Circulatory Care
Circulatory Care: Mechanical Assist Device
Circulatory Precautions
Code Management
Cognitive Restructuring
Cognitive Stimulation
Communication Enhancement: Hearing Deficit
Communication Enhancement: Speech Deficit
Communication Enhancement: Visual Deficit
Complex Relationship Building
Conscious Sedation
Constipation/Impaction Management
Contact Lens Care
Controlled Substance Checking

*From: Nursing Interventions Classification (NIC), (2nd ed.). Copyright© 1995–Iowa Intervention Project. Reprinted with permission.

Coping Enhancement
Cough Enhancement
Counseling
Crisis Intervention
Critical Path Development
Culture Brokerage
Cutaneous Stimulation

Decision-Making Support
Delegation
Delirium Management
Delusion Management
Dementia Management
Developmental Enhancement
Diarrhea Management
Diet Staging
Discharge Planning
Distraction
Documentation
Dressing
Dying Care
Dysreflexia Management
Dysrhythmia Management

Ear Care
Eating Disorders Management
Electrolyte Management
Electrolyte Management: Hypercalcemia
Electrolyte Management: Hyperkalemia
Electrolyte Management: Hypermagnesemia
Electrolyte Management: Hypernatremia
Electrolyte Management: Hyperphosphalemia
Electrolyte Management: Hypocalcemia
Electrolyte Management: Hypolkalemia
Electrolyte Management: Hypomagnesemia
Electrolyte Management: Hyponatremia
Electrolyte Management: Hypophosphatemia
Electrolyte Monitoring
Electronic Fetal Monitoring: Antepartum
Electronic Fetal Monitoring: Intrapartum
Elopement Precautions
Embolus Care: Peripheral
Embolus Care: Pulmonary
Embolus Precautions
Emergency Care
Emergency Cart Check
Emotional Support
Endotracheal Extubation
Energy Management
Enteral Tube Feeding
Environmental Management
Environmental Management: Attachment Process
Environmental Management: Comfort
Environmental Management: Community
Environmental Management: Safety
Environmental Management: Violence Prevention
Environmental Management: Worker Safety
Examination Assistance
Exercise Promotion
Exercise Promotion: Stretching
Exercise Therapy: Ambulation
Exercise Therapy: Balance
Exercise Therapy: Joint Mobility
Exercise Therapy: Muscle Control
Eye Care

Fall Prevention
Family Integrity Promotion
Family Integrity Promotion: Childbearing Family
Family Involvement
Family Mobilization
Family Planning: Contraception
Family Planning: Infertility
Family Planning: Unplanned Pregnancy
Family Process Maintenance
Family Support
Family Therapy
Feeding
Fertility Preservation
Fever Treatment
Fire Setting Precautions
First Aid
Flatulence Reduction
Fluid Management
Fluid Monitoring
Fluid Resuscitation
Fluid/Electrolyte Management
Foot Care

Gastrointestinal Intubation
Genetic Counseling
Grief Work Facilitation
Grief Work Facilitation: Perinatal Death
Grief Work Facilitation

Hair Care
Hallucination Management
Health Care Information Exchange
Health Education
Health Policy Monitoring
Health Screening
Health System Guidance
Heat Exposure Treatment
Heat/Cold Application
Hemodialysis Therapy
Hemodynamic Regulation
Hemorrhage Control
High Risk Pregnancy Care
Home Maintenance Assistance
Hope Instillation
Humor
Hyperglycemia Management
Hypervolemia Management
Hypnosis
Hypoglycemia Management
Hypothermia Treatment
Hypovolemia Management

Immunization/Vaccination Administration
Impulse Control Training
Incident Reporting
Incision Site Care
Infant Care
Infection Control
Infection Control: Intraoperative
Infection Protection
Insurance Authorization
Intracranial Pressure (ICP) Monitoring
Intrapartal Care

Intrapartal Care: High Risk Delivery
Intravenous (IV) Insertion
Intravenous (IV) Therapy
Invasive Hemodynamic Monitoring

Kangaroo Care

Labor Induction
Labor Suppression
Laboratory Data Interpretation
Lactation Counseling
Lactation Suppression
Laser Precautions
Latex Precautions
Learning Facilitation
Learning Readiness Enhancement
Leech Therapy
Limit Setting

Malignant Hyperthermia Precautions
Mechanical Ventilation
Mechanical Ventilatory Weaning
Medication Administration
Medication Administration: Enteral
Medication Administration: Interpleural
Medication Administration: Intraosseous
Medication Administration: Oral
Medication Administration: Parenteral
Medication Administration: Topical
Medication Administration: Ventricular Reservoir
Medication Management
Medication Prescribing
Meditation
Memory Training
Mileu Therapy
Mood Management
Multidisciplinary Care Conference
Music Therapy
Mutual Goal Setting

Nail Care
Neurologic Monitoring
Newborn Care
Newborn Monitoring
Nonnutritive Sucking
Normalization Promotion
Nutrition Management
Nutrition Therapy
Nutritional Counseling
Nutritional Monitoring

Oral Health Maintenance
Oral Health Promotion
Oral Health Restoration
Order Transcription
Organ Procurement
Ostomy Care
Oxygen Therapy

Pain Management
Parent Education: Adolescent
Parent Education: Childbearing Family
Parent Education: Childbearing Family
Pass Facilitation
Patient Contracting
Patient Controlled Analgesia (PCA) Assistance
Patient Rights Protection
Peer Review
Pelvic Floor Exercise
Perineal Care
Peripheral Sensation Management
Peripherally Inserted Central (PIC) Catheter Care
Peritoneal Dialysis Therapy
Phlebotomy: Arterial Blood Sample
Phlebotomy, Blood Unit Acquisition
Phlebotomy: Venous Blood Sample
Phototherapy Neonate
Physical Restraint
Physician Support
Play Therapy
Pneumatic Tourniquet Precautions
Positioning
Positioning: Intraoperative
Positioning: Neurologic
Positioning: Wheelchair
Postanesthesia Care
Postmortem Care
Postpartal Care
Preceptor: Employee
Preceptor: Student
Preconception Counseling
Pregnancy Termination Care
Prenatal Care
Preoperative Coordination
Preparatory Sensory Information
Presence
Pressure Management
Pressure Ulcer Care
Pressure Ulcer Prevention
Product Evaluation
Progressive Muscle Relaxation
Prosthesis Care

Quality Monitoring

Radiation Therapy Management
Rape-Trauma Treatment
Reality Orientation
Recreation Therapy
Rectal Prolapse Management
Referral
Reminiscence Therapy
Reproductive Technology Management
Research Data Collection
Respiratory Monitoring
Respite Care
Resuscitation
Resuscitation: Fetus
Resuscitation: Neonate
Risk Identification
Risk Identification: Childbearing Family
Role Enhancement

Seclusion
Security Enhancement
Seizure Management
Seizure Precautions
Self-Awareness Enhancement
Self-Care Assistance
Self-Care Assistance: Bathing/Hygiene
Self-Care Assistance: Dressing/Grooming
Self-Care Assistance: Feeding
Self-Care Assistance: Toileting
Self-Esteem Enhancement

Self-Modification Assistance
Self-Responsibility Facilitation
Sexual Counseling
Shift Report
Shock Management
Shock Management Cardiac
Shock Management Vasogenic
Shock Management Volume
Shock Prevention
Sibling Support
Simple Guided Imagery
Simple Massage
Simple Relaxation Therapy
Skin Care Topical Treatments
Skin Surveillance
Sleep Enhancement
Smoking Cessation Assistance
Socialization Enhancement
Specimen Management
Spiritual Support
Spining
Staff Supervision
Subarachnoid Hemorrhage Precautions
Substance Use Prevention
Substance Use Treatment
Substance Use Treatment: Alcohol Withdrawal
Substance Use Treatment: Drug Withdrawal
Substance Use Treatment: Overdose
Suicide Prevention
Supply Management
Support Group
Support System Enhancement
Surgical Assistance
Surgical Precautions
Surgical Preparation
Surveillance
Surveillance: Late Pregnancy
Surveillance: Safety
Sustenance Support
Suturing
Swallowing Therapy

Teaching: Disease Process
Teaching: Group
Teaching: Individual
Teaching: Infant Care
Teaching: Preoperative
Teaching: Prescribed Activity/Exercise
Teaching: Prescribed Diet
Teaching: Prescribed Medication
Teaching: Procedure/Treatment
Teaching: Psychomotor Skill
Teaching: Safe Sex
Teaching: Sexuality
Technology Management
Telephone Consultation
Temperature Regulation
Temperature Regulation: Intraoperative
Therapeutic Touch
Therapy Group
Total Parenteral Nutrition (TPN) Administration
Touch
Tract on Immobilization Care
Transcutaneous Electrical Nerve Stimulation (TENS)
Transport
Triage
Truth Telling
Tube Care
Tube Care: Chest
Tube Care: Gastrointestinal
Tube Care: Umbilical Line
Tube Care: Urinary
Tube Care: Ventriculostomy/Lumbar Drain

Ultrasonography: Limited Obstetric
Unilateral Neglect Management
Urinary Bladder Training
Urinary Catheterization
Urinary Catheterization: Intermittent
Urinary Elimination Management
Urinary Habit Training
Urinary Incontinence Care
Urinary Incontinence Care: Enuresis
Urinary Retention Care

Values Clarification
Venous Access Devices (VAD) Maintenance
Ventilation Assistance
Visitation Facilitation
Vital Signs Monitoring

Weight Gain Assistance
Weight Management
Weight Reduction Assistance
Wound Care
Wound Care: Closed Drainage
Wound Irrigation

APPENDIX

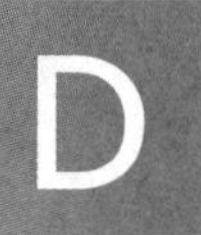

NOC OUTCOMES Approved for Clinical Testing*

abuse cessation
abuse recovery: emotional
abuse recovery: financial
abuse recovery: physical
abuse recovery: protection
abuse recovery: sexual
abusive behavior: self-control
acceptance: health status
adjustment status: life change
aggression control
ambulation: walking
ambulation: wheelchair
anxiety control

balance
blood transfusion reaction control
body image
body positioning: self initiated
bowel elimination

cardiac pump effectiveness
caregiver adaptation to patient institutionalization
caregiver emotional health
caregiver home care readiness
caregiver lifestyle disruption
caregiver performance: direct care
caregiver performance: indirect care
caregiver physical health
caregiver stress
caregiver well-being
caregiver-patient relationship
caregiving endurance potential
child adaptation to hospitalization
circulation status
cognition
cognitive orientation
comfort level
communication
communication: expressive ability
communication: receptive ability
concentration
coping

decision making
distorted thought control

electrolyte & acid/base balance
endurance
energy conservation

family participation in care
fluid balance

grief resolution
growth

health belief: perceived control
health belief: perceived resources
health belief: perceived threat
health beliefs
health beliefs: perceived ability to perform
health orientation
health promoting behavior
health protecting behavior
health seeking behavior
health seeking behavior: adherence
health seeking behavior: compliance
hope
hydration

identity
immobility consequences: physiological
immobility consequences: psycho-cognitive
immune hypersensitivity control
immune status
impulse control
infection status
information processing

joint movement: active
joint movement: passive

knowledge: diet
knowledge: disease process
knowledge: energy conservation
knowledge: health behaviors
knowledge: health resources
knowledge: infection control
knowledge: medication
knowledge: personal safety
knowledge: prescribed activity
knowledge: safe environment
knowledge: substance use control
knowledge: treatment procedure
knowledge: treatment regimen

leisure participation
loneliness

memory
mobility level
mood equilibrium
muscle function

neglect recovery
nutritional status
nutritional status: biochemical measures
nutritional status: body mass
nutritional status: energy
nutritional status: food and fluid intake
nutritional status: nutrient intake

oral health

pain control

---

*Source: ©Nursing-Sensitive Outcomes Classification (NOC), 1995. Reprinted with permission.

pain control behaviors
pain disruptive effects
parent adaptation to child institutionalization
parent home care readiness
parent-infant attachment
participation: health care decisions
peripheral tissue perfusion
physical aging
physical fitness
physical maturation: female
physical maturation: male
play participation

quality of life

respiratory status: gas exchange
respiratory status: ventilation
rest
risk control
risk control: alcohol use
risk control: cardiovascular status
risk control: drug use
risk control: sexually transmitted diseases
risk control: tobacco use
risk control: unintended pregnancy
risk control: vehicle
risk control: weapons
risk control: weight
risk detection

safe environment: fall prevention
safe environment: physical
safe environment: social
safety status: fall injuries
safety status: falls
safety status: personal
self-care: hygiene
self-care: activities of daily living
self-care: bathing
self-care: dressing
self-care: eating
self-care: grooming
self-care: instrumental activities of daily living (IADL)
self-care: non-parenteral medication
self-care: oral hygiene
self-care: parenteral medication
self-care: toileting
self-esteem
self-mutilation control
sleep
social interaction skills
social involvement
social support
spiritual well-being
substance addiction consequences
suicide control
symptom control
symptom control behavior

thermoregulation
thermoregulation: neonate
tissue integrity: skin & mucous membranes
tissue perfusion: abdominal organs
tissue perfusion: cardiac
tissue perfusion: cerebral
tissue perfusion: peripheral
tissue perfusion: pulmonary
transfer performance
treatment behaviors: illness or injury

urinary elimination

vital signs status

well-being
will to live
wound healing: primary intention
wound healing: secondary intention

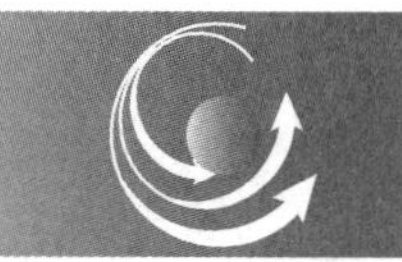

Glossary

Accountable. Being responsible and answerable for something.

Advanced Practice Registered Nurse (APRN). A nurse who, by virtue of credentials (completion of a masters program and certification) has a wide scope of authority to act (may include treating medical problems and prescribing medications).

Affective Domain Outcomes. Measurable goals that deal with changes in attitudes, feelings, or values.

Analyze. To examine and categorize pieces of information to determine where they might fit into the whole picture.

Assessment. The first step of the nursing process, during which you gather and organize data (information) in preparation for the second step, Diagnosis.

Assessment tool. A printed form used to ensure key information is gathered and recorded during Assessment.

Authority. The power or right to act, prescribe, or make a final decision.

Baseline data. Information that describes the status of a problem before treatment begins.

Caring behavior. A way of acting that shows understanding and respect for others' ideals, values, feelings, needs, and desires.

CareMap.™ See Critical pathway.

Case Management. An approach to patient care that aims to improve patient outcomes and satisfaction, while reducing overall cost and length or incidence of hospital stays.

Care Partner. See Unlicensed Assistive Personnel (UAP).

Care variance. See Variance in Care.

Client-centered outcome. A statement describing a measurable behavior of a client, family, or group that reflects the desired result of interventions (that the problem, or problems, are prevented, resolved, or controlled).

Client goal. See Client-centered outcome.

Clinical pathway. See Critical pathway.

Collaborative problem. Potential complications of trauma, disease, or treatment (Carpenito, 1997b).

Cognitive domain outcomes. Measurable goals that deal with acquiring knowledge or intellectual skills.

Competence. The quality of having the necessary knowledge and skill to perform an action in a safe and appropriate manner.

Critical. Characterized by careful and exact evaluation and judgment.

Critical pathway. A standard plan that predicts the course of recovery and day-by-day care required to achieve outcomes for a specific health problem within a specific time frame.

Critical thinking. See Display 1–1, page 17.

Cues. Pieces of information that prompt you to make a judgment

Data. Pieces of information.

Data base assessment. Comprehensive data collected on initial contact with the patient to gain information about all aspects of the patient's health.

Data base form. See Assessment tool.

Defining characteristics. A cluster of cues (signs, symptoms, and risk (related) factors) often associated with a specific nursing diagnosis.

Diagnostic error. When a health problem has been overlooked or incorrectly identified.

Direct care interventions. Actions performed through interaction with patients. Some examples: helping someone out of bed, teaching someone about diabetes.

Discharge goal. A client-centered outcome that describes what the patient will be able to do upon discharge from a facility.

Definitive diagnosis. The most specific, most correct, diagnosis.

Definitive interventions. The most specific treatment required to prevent, resolve, or control a health problem.

Delegation. The transfer of responsibility for the performance of an activity while retaining accountability (ANA, 1993).

Diagnose. To make a judgment and identify a problem or strength based on evidence from an assessment.

Diagnosis. 1) The second step of the nursing process. 2) The *process* of analyzing data and putting related cues together to make judgments about health status. 3) The opinion or judgment that's drawn after the diagnostic process is completed.

Direct data. Information gained directly from the patient.

Diagnostic reasoning. A method of thinking that involves specific, deliberate use of critical thinking to reach conclusions about health status.

Diagnostic statement. A phrase that clearly describes a diagnosis; includes the problem name, etiology, and any evidence confirming the diagnosis.

Empathy. Understanding another's feelings or perceptions, but not sharing the same feelings or point of view (compare with sympathy).

Etiology. Something known to cause a disease. The terms *risk factors and etiology* may be used interchangeably.

Expedite. To accomplish something quickly.

Focus assessment. Data collection that concentrates on gathering more information about a specific problem or condition.

Guidelines. See Display 4–2 on page 115.

Habits of inquiry. Thinking habits that enhance your ability to search for the truth (eg, following rules of logic).

Humanistic. See Caring behavior.

Indicator. See Display 6–3 on page 185.

Indirect care interventions. Actions performed away from the patient, but on behalf of a patient or group of patients. These actions are aimed at management of the health care environment and interdisciplinary collaboration.

Indirect data. Information gained from sources other than the patient (eg, someone's wife).

Inference. How someone perceives or interprets a cue (eg, one person may perceive a person's silence as acceptance, while another may interpret it as defiance).

Intervention. Something done to maximize comfort and human functioning (eg, turning someone every 2 hours is an intervention to maintain skin integrity and assist lung function).

Intuition. Knowing something without having supporting evidence.

Judgment. An opinion that's made after analyzing and synthesizing information.

Life processes. Events or changes that occur during one's lifetime (eg, growing up, aging, maturing, becoming a parent, moving, separations, losses).

Long-term goal. An objective that's expected to be achieved over a relatively long time period, usually weeks or months.

Medical diagnosis. A problem requiring definitive diagnosis by a qualified physician or advanced practice nurse.

Medical domain. Activities and actions a physician is legally qualified to perform or prescribe.

Medical orders. Interventions ordered by a physician or advanced practice nurse to treat a medical problem.

Medical process. The method physicians use to expedite diagnosis and treatment of diseases or trauma. The medical process focuses mainly on problems with structure and function of organs or systems.

Multidisciplinary plan. A plan that's developed collaboratively by key members of the health-care team (eg, nursing, physical therapy, medicine, and others).

Need. A requirement that, if fulfilled, reduces stress and promotes a sense of adequacy and well-being.

Nurse extender. See Unlicensed Assistive Personnel (UAP).

Nursing Assistant. See Unlicensed Assistive Personnel (UAP).

Nursing Diagnosis. A clinical judgment about an individual, family, or community response to actual or potential health problems and life processes. Nursing diagnoses provide the basis for selection of nursing interventions to achieve outcomes for which the nurse is accountable (NANDA, 1990).

Nursing diagnoses are often called *human responses* because we as nurses focus on how people *are responding* to changes in health or life circumstances. For example, how they're responding to illness, or to becoming a parent.

Nursing domain. Activities and actions a nurse is legally qualified to perform or prescribe.

Nurse-prescribed intervention. An action a nurse may legally order or initiate independently. (Carpenito, 1997b).

Nursing Process. A systematic, outcome-oriented method that nurses use to expedite diagnosis and treatment of actual and potential health problems.

Objective data. Information, that's measurable and observable (eg, blood pressure, pulse, diagnostic studies).

Outcome. The result of prescribed interventions. Usually refers to the *desired result* of interventions (ie, that the problem is prevented, resolved, or controlled), and includes a specific time frame for when the goal is expected to be achieved.

Outcome based practice. Healthcare practice that's focused on achieving desired results efficiently (ie, that patients achieve the expected results of care).

Patient Care Technician. See Unlicensed Assistive Personnel (UAP).

Performance Assessment and Improvement. See Display 6–3 on page 000.

Physician-prescribed (or Delegated) intervention. An action ordered by a physician for a nurse or another health care professional to perform. (Carpenito, 1997b).

Policies. See Display 4–2 on page 115.

PQI. See Display 6–3 on page 185.

Proactive. A way of thinking and behaving that accepts responsibility for one's actions and takes initiative to plan ahead to anticipate and prevent problems before they happen. (comes from act before).

Procedures. See Display 4–2 on page 115.

Protocols. See Display 4–2 on page 115.

Prognosis. The predicted course or outcome of disease or trauma.

Psychomotor outcomes. Measurable goals that deal with acquiring skills that require deliberate, specific muscle coordination to perform an activity (eg, walking with crutches).

QA (Quality Assessment). See Display 6–3 on page 185.

QI (Quality Improvement). See Display 6–3 on page 185.

Qualified. Having the knowledge, skill, and authority to perform an action.

Quality. See Display 6–3 on page 185.

Quality care. Cost-effective healthcare that increases the probability of achieving desired results and decreases the probability of undesired results.

Related factor. Something known to be *associated with* a specific diagnosis. See also *Risk factor*.

Risk factor. Something known to cause or *contribute to* a specific problem. For example, *decreased vision* is a related factor of *Risk for Injury*.

Risk (potential) diagnosis. A health problem which may develop if preventive actions aren't taken.

Sign. Objective data that indicate an abnormality.

Subjective data. Information the patient or client tells the nurse during Assessment (usually charted as "Patient states . . .").

Short-term goal. A client-centered outcome that's achieved as a stepping stone to reaching a long-term goal.

Standards. See Display 4–2 on page 115.

Standard Care Plan. See Display 4–2 on page 115.

Standard of Care. See Display 4–2 on page 115.

Standard of Practice. See Display 4–2 on page 115.

Standards of Professional Performance. See Display 4–2 on page 115.

Sympathy. Sharing the same feelings as another (compare with empathy).

Symptom. Subjective data that indicate an abnormality.

Syndrome diagnosis. A cluster of nursing diagnoses often associated with a specific situation or event (Carpenito, 1997b).

Unlicensed Assistive Personnel (UAP). Someone without a license to practice nursing who is hired to assist nurses in care delivery. These individuals may have a variety of job titles (eg, nursing assistant, nurse extender, care partner, patient care technician) and have varied job descriptions and capabilities.

Variance in care. When a patient hasn't achieved activities or outcomes by the time frame noted on a critical path. A variance in care triggers additional assessment to determine whether the delay is justified or whether actions need to be taken to improve the patient's likelihood of achieving the outcome. (Iyer, 1994).

Validation. The process of making sure the information you collect is factual and complete.

Wellness diagnosis. A clinical judgment about an individual, family, or community in transition from a specific level of wellness to a higher level of wellness (NANDA, 1990).

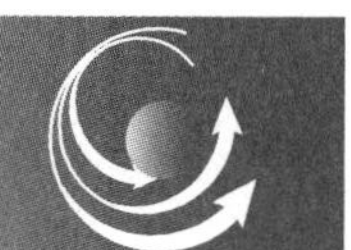

Index

Note: Page numbers followed by *f* indicate figures; page numbers followed by *t* indicate tables.

A

D

E

F

G

H

I

J

K

L

M

N

O

Q

R

S